AF413306

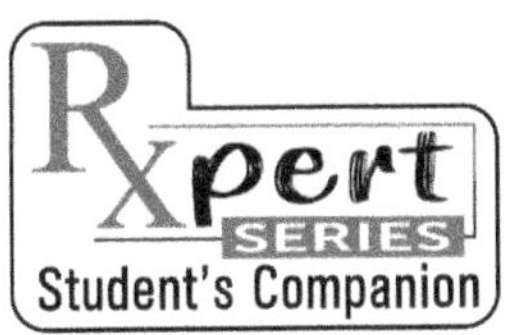

Concepts of Social Pharmacy

Komal Sharma M.Pharm, Ph.D.

Professor in Pharmacology,
Bhupal Nobles' College of Pharmacy
BN University, Udaipur.

Neelam Singla M. Pharm., Ph.D

Professor in Pharmaceutical Chemistry
Suresh Gyan Vihar University
Jaipur (Rajasthan).

Abhishek Tiwari M. Pharm., Ph.D.

Professor
Department of Pharmaceutical Chemistry,
Pharmacy Academy, IFTM University,
Lodhipur Rajput, Delhi Road, NH-24,
Moradabad, U.P. 244102.

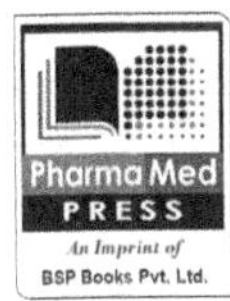

PharmaMed Press

An imprint of BSP Books Pvt. Ltd.

4-4-309/316, Giriraj Lane,
Sultan Bazar, Hyderabad - 500 095.

Concepts of Social Pharmacy

by **Komal Sharma, Neelam Singla and Abhishek Tiwari**

© 2023, *by Publisher*

All rights reserved.

Disclaimer: The authors and the publishers have taken due care to provide the authentic, reliable and up to date information related to the subject. However, neither the authors nor the publisher shall be responsible for any liability for any damage caused as a result of use of this book. The respective user must check the accuracy from other sources too.

Published by

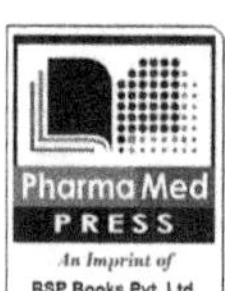

PharmaMed Press

An imprint of BSP Books Pvt. Ltd.

4-4-309/316, Giriraj Lane, Sultan Bazar, Hyderabad - 500 095.
Phone: 040-23445688; Fax: 91+40-23445611
E-mail: info@pharmamedpress.net
www.bspbooks.net/www.pharmamedpress.net

ISBN: 978-93-95039-50-5 (Hardback)

PREFACE

Social pharmacy as a concept emphasizes that the practice of pharmacy should extend beyond academics, research, industry, and drug distribution, and calls for social interaction between the general population and pharmacists. The objective of the social pharmacy course is to demonstrate how pharmacists may play a vital role in achieving public health goals

It inspired us to write a complete, informative book for the students and develop their interest in this subject. The book provides a comprehensive and simple guide in areas such as preventive health care, food and nutrition, national health programs and policies, epidemiology, pharmacoeconomics, and disaster management.

This being the first edition, may have certain errors. We welcome the corrections and suggestions for future editions. Kindly send your feedback at

komalsharmagautam@gmail.com

neelams.singla@gmail.com

abhishekt1983@gmail.com

- Authors

Contents

Chapter 4

Introduction to Microbiology and Common Microorganisms

Chapter 5

Introduction to Health Systems and all Ongoing National Health Programs in India

Chapter 6

Role of Pharmacist in Disaster Management

Chapter 7

Pharmaeconomics

CHAPTER 1

Introduction to Social Pharmacy

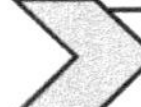

1.1 Introduction

The pharmaceutical sector in India is one of the major pillars of the country's healthcare system and has made significant contributions to the population's health and well-being by providing access to low-cost, high-quality medications. The main components are:

- Pharmaceutical industry (Manufacturers of medicines)

- Supply and distribution (Wholesaler and retailers of medicines and other medical products)

- Facilities (All institutions where healthcare is provided through the healthcare workforce i.e. hospitals, nursing homes, clinics)

LEARNING OBJECTIVES

This chapter aims to provide students with an understanding of the following topics:

- Definition and Scope. Social Pharmacy as a discipline and its scope in improving public health. Role of Pharmacists in Public Health.

- Concept of Health -WHO Definition, various dimensions, determinants, and health indicators.

- National Health Policy – Indian perspective

- Public and Private Health System in India, National Health Mission

- Introduction to Millennium Development Goals, Sustainable Development Goals, FIP Development Goals

- Healthcare workforce (All people who deliver or assist in the delivery of healthcare services mainly doctors, nurses, medical lab technicians, and to some extent pharmacists)

The pharmacy practice in India has remained focused largely on the products (drugs) oriented roles such as manufacturing, selling, dispensing medications, record keeping, etc. The sector is promoted by various Government initiatives at different levels

At the Industry level, it is done by promoting pharmaceutical manufacturing industries in different states to increase access to medicines. It is done by incentivizing through:

- Competitive land rates

- Low resource costs like water, electricity, and civil infrastructure

- Lower cost of production machinery

- Tax exemption

At the Policy level, the National Pharmaceutical Pricing Authority regulates and monitors the price and distribution of essential medicines.

At the Hospital level, access to free medicines is provided by

- Direct procurement from manufacturers and supplying to Government hospitals.

- Health insurance coverage through schemes (Ayushman Bharat).

- Government-approved Jan Aushidhi stores to sell affordable medicines.

As a result of these government programs and systems, the Indian Pharmaceutical industry has shown robust growth and caters to the medicine demand of millions of people through its extensive distribution system.

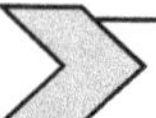 ## 1.2   Social Pharmacy as a Discipline

To date, the scope of pharmacists/pharmacy professionals is limited to drug manufacturing, sales, and research but underutilized in public or social health discourse.

What is Public Health: According to World Health Organization (WHO), public health refers to organized measures to **prevent disease, promote health and prolong life** among the population as a whole.

Social pharmacy is introduced to bring public health education to the pharmacy profession.

Social pharmacy is an effort to maintain the relevance of pharmacy concerning societal and population needs. *It is defined as the discipline dealing with the role of medicines from social, scientific, and humanistic perspectives i.e. all social aspects that impact or influence the use of medication.*

Social pharmacy as a concept aims to highlight that the practice of pharmacy should be seen beyond academia, research, industry, and distribution, and requires social interaction between the general public and pharmacists. The focus of social pharmacy is on improving the health of the population through the use of medicines and healthcare services. It could be accomplished by providing the students with proper knowledge and resources in the following areas:

- Public health and national health programs

- Preventive healthcare

- Food and nutrition-related health issues

- Health education and health promotion
- Roles and responsibilities of pharmacists in public health

Scope of Social Pharmacy

This scope of social pharmacy is to impart basic knowledge on the concepts of:

- ➢ **Preventive care**: It is the prevention of disease and health promotion rather than the diagnosis and treatment of diseases through national public health initiatives e.g. vaccination, family planning, mother and child care, breastfeeding promotion, environmental pollution due to pharmaceuticals, the social impact of drug abuse.

- ➢ **Epidemiology**: Epidemiology is the scientific study of the spread and control of disease in the human population e.g. communicable diseases (chickenpox, whooping cough, covid 19, etc) The aim is to use knowledge of cause and effect to break links between disease and its causes and to improve health.

- ➢ **Nutrition and health**: Nutrition, healthy diets, and food quality have a strong relationship with the prevention of illness and disease. Studying the impact of nutrition on public health can improve the health of the population.

- ➢ **Public health Programmes:** These are the measures taken by the government to control and eradicate diseases that cause mortality and improve the health of people e.g. national programs related to mother and child care, immunization, control of nutritional deficiency disorders, etc. Pharmacists must have knowledge about various health programs as he plays a major role in their execution to strengthen the health system.

- ➢ **Pharmacoeconomics:** It is a branch of health economics related to the cost evaluation of medicines. The knowledge helps to design strategies for cost-effective treatments.

Role of Pharmacist in Public Health

- ➢ The health and health outcomes of a community depend on the availability, accessibility, and quality of health workers.

- ➢ Pharmacists are considered important members of this health workforce involved in the overall well-being of the general population.

- ➢ They operate in a variety of contexts, including clinical/hospital, community, industrial, policy, program management, education, and research.

Pharmacists can be part of the public health outreach programs through:

1. **Medication therapy management (MTM):** Mismanagement of medications and medication-related problems are serious issues for public health. It can be addressed through medication therapy management. Pharmacists can be an integral part of the healthcare team by participating in the following activities:

➤ Conducting a comprehensive review of patients' medications including over-the-counter and herbal products and identifying the mismanagement of medications such as the misuse, duplication, and/or unnecessary use of medications.

➤ Detecting the need of medication for an untreated or inappropriately managed medical condition.

➤ Providing medication-related education, consultation, and advice to patients, their families, and caregivers to help ensure appropriate medication utilization.

2. **Cost management:** The cost of healthcare has increased due to the growing burden of disease. Pharmacists with pharmacoeconomics knowledge may identify, evaluate, and compare the price of various pharmacotherapies or services and significantly lower the treatment cost.

3. **Participating in National health programs:** Pharmacists' involvement in HIV/AIDS prevention and control; and tuberculosis control programs have recently rolled out. With detailed knowledge about National health missions and programs, pharmacists can "actively participate in all the national health programs", through involvement in health awareness campaigns run by the government of India and "communicate and cooperate effectively with the other members of the health care team". e.g. leprosy and vector-borne disease control, mental health, deafness and blindness control, pulse polio, universal immunization, health care of the elderly, and tobacco control programs

4. **Preventive care:** From a public health perspective, Pharmacists can provide **preventative care** via immunizations (vaccines) or by informing individuals on how best to self-manage certain habits the cessation of smoking. These initiatives will help to minimize health costs and save people from infectious diseases.

5. **Participation in policy-making decisions:** Pharmacists that are educated in epidemiology can study medication use, safety, and efficacy in various population groups, critically evaluate the benefits and risks of medications over time, and provide that information to regulatory agencies and healthcare professionals. The analysis of 'big data' by epidemiologists

generates new plans and strategies to improve clinical health and making policy decisions regarding medicine use.

6. **Nutritional counselor/educator:** Pharmacists can provide nutritional counselling. For example:

➢ Good dietary choices and lifestyle strategies for disease prevention e.g. type 2 diabetes can be controlled by a low carbohydrate diet.

➢ Assessing possible drug-nutrient interactions, drug-food interactions, and, drug-drug interactions that may be detrimental to nutritional support therapy.

➢ Selection and use of oral nutritional supplements.

7. **Disaster management:** Pharmacists are the most common health care professionals. Pharmacist's centralized position in the community makes them valuable during disasters to provide healthcare continuity. Apart from dispensing medicine, pharmacists have proven to be an accessible resource for health and medication information. There are many functions of public health that can benefit from pharmacists' unique expertise that may include pharmacotherapy, access to care and prevention services.

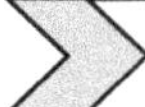 ## 1.3   Concept of Health

Health is viewed from various perspectives therefore different definitions of health are available in literature today. Some of the perceptions include:

➢ The oldest known definition of health is **that health is the absence of disease.**

➢ The ancient Indians and Greeks view health as harmony i.e. being at peace with oneself, with the community, with God, and with the cosmos (**Park, 2009**).

➢ Health is a state of vibrancy, physical strength, and the ability to perform the needed task.

➢ Health has also been conceived as the condition under which the individual can mobilize all his resources, intellectual, emotional, and physical, for an optimum living (**Pulga, 1983**).

➢ Health is the ability to function effectively within a given environment (**Schiffer, 1980**).

One common factor in these definitions and concepts of health is that health is portrayed as a positive phenomenon associated with longevity, peace, soundness of mind, and happiness. In recent years new thinking about health emerged which can be summarized as follows:

➤ Health is a **fundamental human right** and should be available to all.

➤ Productive life is rooted in health and not based on medical expenditure.

➤ Health is inter-sectoral and cannot be achieved through a single sector effort.

➤ Health is a vital component of development and therefore a constituent of Sustainable Development Goals.

➤ Health is a multi-level responsibility carried out at the individual, state, and international levels.

➤ Health and the maintenance of health constitute a major social investment.

➤ Health is a global social goal.

WHO: The World Health Organization (WHO) is a specialized agency of the **United Nations** responsible for international public health. The main objective is the attainment of the highest possible level of health by all people.

> The concept of health developed by the World Health Organization (WHO) in1947 states that health is "a state of complete physical, mental, and social well-being and not merely the absence of disease or infirmity."

This includes the following types of health:

1. **Physical health** can be defined as the proper functioning of all the external and internal parts and organs of the person's body which allows the person to perform the daily task normally without any limitation.

2. **Good mental health** means a person should be able to understand the potential, can manage general and normal life stresses and may be able to participate in society and to work effectively.

3. **Social health** can be defined as how the person can interact with people for example friends, family, and society. When a person is socially healthy, it helps him or her to develop relationships with other people in society. It also helps people in their careers and enables them to live independently in their life. Ensuring that all aspects of one's health are functioning well will develop a better sense of overall well-being.

Well-being is explained as a positive feeling that a person experiences in the absence of ill health. It is connected with the accomplishment of an individual's own goals and by achieving these goals, the person feels well and good.

Evolution of the WHO concept of Health

Over time the definition of health has changed to reflect the inter-sectoral nature of health. Health is multi-dimensional, spanning beyond the three dimensions contained in the World Health Organization's definition of health (physical, mental and social) to encompass dimensions such as spiritual, emotional, vocational, and political dimensions, etc.

Dimensions of Health

All eight dimensions of health are proposed that interact and influence each other. Each dimension contributes in its own way to our wellness or quality of life. These are divided into internal and external factors.

Internal Factors: Physical, emotional, mental, and spiritual. They relate to the internal state of one's body, mind, and spirit.

External factors: Environmental, social, financial, and occupational factors relate to the way you interact with the external world and how it influences you.

1. Physical Dimension (the state of your body):

- This is based on the biological concept of health and implies a situation where the body's cells, organs, and systems are **functioning at optimum capacity and are in harmony with the rest of the body**.

- Signs of physical health include; good appetite, bright eyes, good complexion, lustrous hair, and regular bladder and bowel movement among others.

- Physical health can be measured in modern medicine using self-assessment of overall health, investigation of symptoms of illness and associated risk factors, medication and use of medical services, etc.

2. Mental Dimension (the state of your mind and brain):

- The mental dimension of health denotes the ability to respond appropriately to experiences of life and not the mere absence of mental illness.

- A person with mental health will exhibit sense of purpose and will relate with others harmoniously.

- Mental health refers to maintaining a state of equilibrium between the individual and the world around him.

- Psychological factors can generate other types of illnesses other than mental illness, such as hypertension and peptic ulcer among others.

3. Social Dimension (the state of your support system and satisfaction with the roles you play):

➤ The social dimension of health originated from the concept of the human being as a part of a family and also part of the larger society where a person lives and relates with others.

➤ Social health emerges from a positive environment (focusing on financial and residential matters) and a positive human environment (social network of the individual).

➤ It portrays maintaining healthy relationships, enjoying being with others, developing friendships and intimate relations, caring about others, and contributing to your community (social networks) and favorable economic conditions.

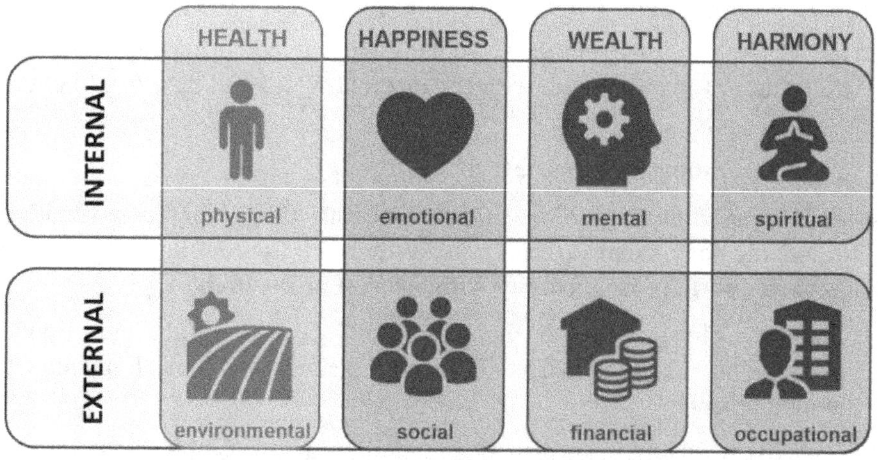

Figure 1.1 Eight dimensions of wellness

4. Spiritual dimension (the state of living with meaning and purpose):

➤ The spiritual dimension of health focuses on that part of the individual which strives for finding purpose, value, and meaning in his/her life.

➤ The elements of the spiritual dimension of health comprise of integrity, principles, ethics, purpose in life and commitment to a higher being.

➤ The holistic concept of health gives serious consideration to the spiritual dimension for its role in health and disease. Anyone who experiences spiritual uneasiness or who is not spiritually at peace is not likely to put up appropriate behavior that reflects wholeness.

5. Emotional dimension (the state of feeling):

➤ This dimension considers the influence of the emotional aspect of a human being on his health.

> Though closely related to mental health, it differentiates as the emotional dimension aligns with feelings and the mental to cognition

> Emotional disturbances will affect the individual's response and adaptation to his environment and the way he relates to other persons around him.

6. **Occupational or Vocational Dimension (Your job and career satisfaction):**

> It is a new dimension ascribed to health and it focuses on the vocational aspect of life.

> Work is part of human existence and plays a role in promoting physical and mental health.

> Preparing for and participating in work and the achievement of goals brings about self-realization, satisfaction, and self-esteem.

> This dimension is appreciated when there is a life event that reverses this process such as losing a job which can result in a crisis for the person concerned.

7. **Environmental dimension**

> The environmental dimension encompasses a healthy relationship with the earth and its resources and a healthy relationship with your surroundings.

> It means being intentional about Protecting oneself from environmental hazards, such as noise, chemicals, pollution, and ultraviolet radiation.

8. **Non-medical dimensions of health (Financial wellbeing)** :

They contribute to a level of health that allows for socio-economic productivity among persons. These dimensions include:

> Financial status affects health to a large extent as people of lower socio-economic dimensions (occupation, economic level) lack proper nutrition, live in unhygienic conditions, and are not able to afford the expense of health services.

> Cultural dimension (family and cultural belief, religious belief).

> Educational dimension (access to education).

> Nutritional dimension (access to healthy food).

> Curative dimension (therapy to cure the patient).

> Preventive dimension (measures to prevent healthy people from becoming ill).

Outcomes of the Wellness (Health) Dimensions

The eight factors influencing one's wellness can further be divided into four pairs. When each pair is seen in its totality and is optimized, it leads to the fulfilment of the desired outcome. The conceptualization is:

- When the **physical** and **environmental** pair are optimized, they lead to **HEALTH**

- When the **emotional** and **social** pair are optimized, they lead to **HAPPINESS.**

- When the **mental** and **financial** pair are optimized, they lead to **WEALTH**

- When the **spiritual** and **occupation** pair are optimized, they lead to **HARMONY**

Determinants of Health: Health includes more than just health care. At every stage of life, health is determined by complex interactions between social and economic factors, the physical environment, and individual behaviour. They do not exist in isolation from each other.

To a large extent, factors such as where we live, the state of our environment, genetics, our income, education level, our relationships with friends and family, and access to healthcare services all have considerable impacts on health. Research shows there are 4 broad factors (other than genetics) that influence our health.

The Drivers of Health

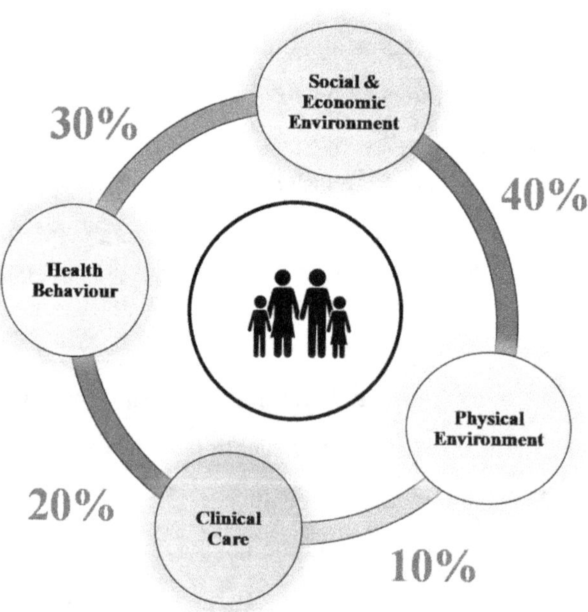

Figure 1.2 Drivers of health

The determinants of health and their relative contribution

- Social and economic environment (40%)
- Physical environment (10%)
- Person's characteristics and behaviors (30%)
- Clinical care (20%)

1. **The Social & Economic Environment:** Our social and economic environments influence health. The social and economic environment includes access to quality education, job opportunities, safe neighborhoods, social support, and healthy foods

   Education: A person's education and income are the greatest predictors of their health.

   - Individuals with higher levels of education and income tend to live longer, healthier lives. This relationship exists at both the individual and community levels.
   - Illiteracy coincides with poverty, malnutrition, and ill-health

   Occupation: Suitable and productive employment promotes health as

   - Proper employment generates income and raises economic status which in turn promotes health and education of family
   - Job satisfaction contributes to mental health and well being

   Economic Status: It is measured as GNP (Gross National Product) i.e. average income of the citizen of a country) and tells the economic status of a country It includes purchasing power, the standard of living family size, and attention towards health care.

   - Economic progress is a major factor in reducing morbidity, increasing life expectancy, and improving quality of life.
   - On the contrary, affluence can lead to a high incidence of diabetes, obesity, and coronary heart disease in upper socio-economic groups.

   Political System: Political system can shape the health of the people in the country through:

   - Creating affordable and available healthcare facilities for different segments of society.
   - Resource allocation for the health sector.
   - Environment protection.
   - Choice of technology.

2. **Clinical or Healthcare Services:** Clinical care refers to any interaction with the health care system, ranging from preventive activities like vaccines for prospective mothers, infants, and children and general screening programs for the treatment of particular diseases and conditions, blindness and cancer due to preventive causes, etc. It can occur in a variety

of settings, including outpatient clinics, hospitals, public health departments, long-term care facilities, and in some cases our own homes. Effective health care should be accessible, affordable, timely, and of high quality.

3. **Life Style or health behavior:** These are the choices we make that affect the length and quality of our lives.

   - Some of the significant health behaviours are smoking, physical activity, and diet. All 3 affect a person's risk for developing diabetes, cardiovascular disease, cancer, obesity, and other chronic illnesses.

   - Behavioral change in these 3 areas can seriously affect our health outcomes and quality of life. Health behaviours are a personal choice and certain health behaviour promote health e.g. eating a nutritional diet, enough physical activity, and enough sleep.

4. **Physical Environment:** It encompasses the natural and built environments including transportation systems, buildings, and public resources.

People's school, work, and home environments have a direct effect on their health and also influence their health behaviours. For example, access to sidewalks, parks, and playgrounds offers opportunities for physical activity, while exposure to pollution or unsafe drinking water contributes to health conditions like asthma and waterborne illness.

5. **Genetics:** Inheritance or Genetics plays a part in determining lifespan, healthiness, and the likelihood of developing certain illnesses. Several diseases are known to be of genetic origin e.g. epilepsy, cancer, diabetes, mental retardation, and metabolic problems.

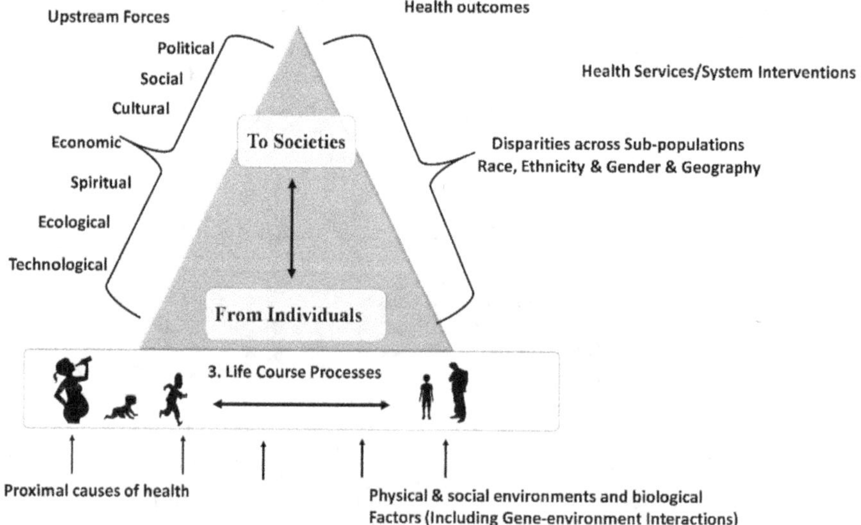

Figure 1.3 Determinants of health in the society

Health Indicators

A health indicator is an estimated measurement of a given health dimension in a target population. The collected data after analysis become a synonym for "indicator of the population's health," rather than "indicator of individual health." and address the following concerns

- How healthy is the community?
- Is our community in balance?
- What factors affect the health of the population?
- Are programs or services working?
- Are we moving towards or away from the vision of health?

Significance of health indicators: The health indicators are useful in

- Measuring the health status of a community and also comparing the health status of one country with another.
- Estimating healthcare needs and allocation of resources.
- Monitoring and evaluation of health services activities and programs and measuring the extent to which the objectives and targets of a healthcare program have been achieved.

Classification of Health Indicators: Health indicators are subdivided into the following:

A. Health Status Indicators:

1. **Mortality indicators:** Mortality data may provide a crude but simple way to assess health conditions. The source of information can be a death certificate where the cause of death is written. The specific indicators are:

   - ***Crude Death Rate:*** *it* is defined as the number of death per thousand populations per year in a given community. It is a good tool for assessing overall health improvement in a population.

     Number of deaths during the year × 1000/ Mid-year population

   - **Life expectancy:** Life expectancy at birth is the average number of years a person is likely to live. Currently, in India, it is 69.66 years.

   - **Age-specific death rates:** The total number of deaths occurring in a specific age group of the population for example 15 to 20 years in a defined area during a specific period per 1000 estimated total population of the same group.

   - **Infant mortality rate:** It is the ratio of deaths under 1 year of age in a given year to the total number of live births in the same year it is expressed as the rate per thousand life birth. It is one of the most universally accepted indicators.

Number of deaths under 1 year of age in the given year × 1000/ Total number of live births in the same year

➤ **Child mortality rate:** It is related to the overall health status in the early childhood mortality rate 1 to 4 years

*Number of deaths at 1- 4 years of age in the given year × 1000/ Children in that age group at the midpoint of the yea*r

➤ **Under 5 proportionate mortality rate**: It is the proportion of deaths occurring in the under 5 age group.

Number of deaths under 5 years of age in the given year × 1000/ Total number of deaths during the same period

➤ **Maternal Mortality rate (MMR)**: It is the annual number of female deaths per 1,00,000 live births from any cause related to pregnancy, childbirth, or its management.

Table 1.1 Health indicators

Health status indicators (Disease specific)	Determinants of health (Biological risk factors and health behavior	Health system indicators
• Mortality indicators • Morbidity indicators • Disability rates	• Nutritional status indicator • Social & mental health indicators • Environmental indicators • Socio-economic indicators • Indicators of quality of life	• Health care delivery indicators • Utilization rates • Healthypolicy indicators

2. **Morbidity Indicators:** These indicators are used to supplement mortality data. The following morbidity rates are used for assessing ill health in the community:

➤ **Incidence and prevalence:** The number of new cases occurring in a defined population during a specified period.

Incidence = Number of new cases of a specific disease during a given period × 1000/ the population at risk during that period

➤ **Prevalence:** The total number of all individuals who have the disease at a particular time divided by the population having that disease during that period.

➤ **Notification rates:** Reporting to public authorities of diseases e.g. Polio, TB

➤ The attendance rate at OPDs

➤ Admission, readmission, and discharge rates Spells of sickness

3. **Disability Rates**: The following indicators have been used:

> **DALY (Disability-Adjusted Life Years):** It measures the disease burden in the population and takes into account premature death along with years lost due to disability caused by disease or injury.

> **PYL (Potential years of life lost):** It measures the impact of premature death on the population. It is the sum of the years that people would have lived, had they experienced normal life expectancy.

B. Indicators based upon Determinants of Health

1. **Nutritional Status Indicators:** It includes:

> Anthropometric measurement of pre-school children e,g. weight and height.

> Height of children at school entry.

> Prevalence of low birth weight (less than 2.5 Kg).

2. **Social & Mental Health Indicators:**

> Suicide, homicide, other acts of violence, road traffic accidents e.g. alcohol and drug abuse are examples.

> These indicators provide a guide to social action for improving the health.

3. **Environmental Indicators:**

> These reflect the quality of the physical and biological environment.

> The proportion of the population having access to safe water.

> The proportion of the population having access to sanitation facilities.

> Indicators relating to pollution of air and water, radiation, solid wastes, noise.

4. **Socio-Economic Indicators:**

These indicators do not directly measure health but they are of great importance in the interpretation of the indicators of health care e.g.

> Rate of population decrease

> Per capita income

> Level of unemployment

> Dependency ratio

> Literacy rate

> Family size

> Housing

5. **Quality of Life Indicators**: These indicators are difficult to measure so expressed as the index value

   ➤ **PQLI** (Physical quality of life): It is calculated by the average of three indicators infant mortality, life expectancy at age 1, and literacy.

   ➤ **Human Development Index**: It combines longevity, education, and gross national income.

C. Health System Indicators

1. **Health care delivery indicators:** These indicators reflect the distribution of health resources.

   ➤ Doctor: Population ratio, Doctor: Nurse ratio

   ➤ Population: Bed ratio

   ➤ Population per health sub-center

2. **Utilization indicators**: express the proportion of the population in need of healthcare services e.g.

   ➤ The proportion of infants who are fully immunized

   ➤ Percentage of the population using various methods of family planning

   ➤ Average daily inpatient cases

3. **Health Policy Indicators:** Important indicator of political commitment is the "Allocation of adequate resources"

   ➤ The proportion of GNP spent on health services

   ➤ The proportion of GNP spent on health-related activities

   ➤ The proportion of total health resources devoted to primary health care

Uses of Health Indicators:

1. **Addressing unmet needs**: Health indicators can be used to describe health care needs in a population, and the disease burden in specific population groups. The description of a population's health needs can guide decisions about the extent and nature of unmet needs, the inputs needed to address the problem, and the groups that should receive the greatest attention, among other functions.

2. **Forecast or prognosis:** Health indicators can be used to anticipate results about the state of health of a population or a group of patients (prognosis). These indicators are used to forecast disease burdens in populations, and disease outbreaks, thereby helping to prevent epidemics.

3. **Explanation:** Health indicators can facilitate an understanding of why some individuals in a population are healthy and others are not by

indicators about social determinants of health, such as gender roles and norms, ethnicity, income, and social support

4. **System management and quality improvement**: The production and regular monitoring of health indicators can also provide feedback to improve decision-making in various systems and sectors.

5. **Evaluation**: Health indicators can show the results of health interventions. The monitoring of such indicators can detect the impact of health policies, programs, services, and actions.

6. **Advocacy**: Indicators can serve as tools to support or oppose particular ideas and ideologies in different historical and cultural contexts.

7. **Accountability**. Health indicators can provide needed information on risks, disease and mortality patterns, and health-related trends over time for governments, health professionals, international organizations, and civil society which is necessary to monitor a population's health situation and trends.

8. **Research:** Observation of the distribution of health indicators can generate a hypothesis to explain observed trends and discrepancies.

9. **Measure gender gaps**: Gender-sensitive indicators measure gaps between men and women resulting from differences or inequalities in gender roles, norms, and relations.

The indicators used in public health are **to drive decision-making for health**. The ultimate objective is to improve the health of the population and reduce unjust and preventable inequalities.

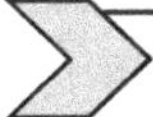 ## 1.4   National Health Policy-Indian Perspective

A healthy population is the goal of every country. No country can afford to neglect the issue of health, as the health status of an individual plays an important role in human capital generation. Policies serve the purpose of providing specific guidelines which help in guiding the intervention in the area of public health.

Policy: Policy is a system, which provides the logical framework and rationality of decision-making for the achievement of defined goals.

Health Policy

➤ The health policy of a nation is its strategy for controlling and optimizing the social uses of its health knowledge and health resources.

➤ It refers to decisions, plans, and actions that are undertaken to achieve specific health care goals within society.

Background

> Initial systematic efforts to provide health care in India were in accordance with five-year plans as well as recommendations of high-level committees such as the Bhore Committee, Sokhey committee, Mudailar committee, etc.

> The joint WHO – UNICEF international conference in 1978 at Alma Ata (USSR) commented that "The existing gross inequalities in the status of health of people particularly between developed and developing countries as well as within the country is politically, socially and economically unacceptable."

> So, the Alma Ata Declaration called on all governments to formulate National Health Policies according to their circumstances and to launch and sustain primary health care as a part of the national health system.

National Health Policy-1983: After 30 years of independence, the Ministry of Health & Family Welfare, Government of India, introduced its first national health policy (NHP) in 1983. NHP-1983 proposed 'State as a service provider' and 'public provisioning as a model of service delivery.

The aim of the NHP- 1983 with its main focus on the provision of primary health care to all was to achieve **'Health for all by 2000 AD'.** Policy focused on primary health care and equitable access to health services.

The policy stressed the need of establishing comprehensive (that includes everything) primary health care services to reach the population in the remote areas of the country.

India failed to achieve the goal of 'Health for all by 2000 AD' due to slow socio-economic development, insufficient political commitment to the implementation of health for all, and the continuing low status of women. Pollution, poor food safety, and lack of water supply and sanitation also added to the failure of the policy.

National Health Policy 2002: In light of the change in the epidemiological profile of the country, a revised health policy with a major focus to tackle health inequalities and achieve better health care and unmet goals had been brought out by the Government of India- National Health Policy 2002.

Objectives of National Health Policy 2002 were:

> To achieve an acceptable standard of good health for the Indian Population.

> To decentralize the public health system by upgrading infrastructure in existing institutions.

> To ensure more equitable access to health services across the social and geographical regions of India.

➤ To enhance the contribution of the private sector in providing health services for people who can afford to pay.

➤ To give primacy to prevention and first-line curative initiatives.

➤ To emphasize on rational use of drugs.

➤ To increase access to tried systems of Traditional Medicine.

Policy directions of NHP, 2002 resulted in interventions like National Rural Health Mission (NRHM, 2005) and National Urban Health Mission (NUHM, 2013). Both the programs were merged under **National Health Mission** in 2013. Though National health policy 2002 succeeded in eliminating polio but failed to eradicate persisting challenges such as inadequate health services, and low public spending on the healthcare system forces people into poverty to access healthcare.

Table 1.2 Goals of National Health Policy 2002, to be achieved by 2015

Goals of National Health Policy 2022

S. No.	Goal	Year
1)	Eradicate Polio and Yaws	2005
2)	Eliminate leprosy	2005
3)	Established and integrated system of surveillance, National health accounts and health statistics	2005
4)	Increase state sector health spending from 5.5 % to 7 % of the budget.	2005
5)	Achieve zero level growth of HIV/AIDS	2007
6)	Eliminate Kala-Azar	2010
7)	Reduce mortality by 50 %on account of TB, Malaria and other vector& water borne diseases.	2010
8)	Reduce prevalence of blindness to 0.5%	2010
9)	Reduce IMR to 30/1000 and MMR to 100/Lakh	2010
10)	Increase utilization of public health facilities from current level of 20% to 75 %.	2010
11)	Increase health Expenditure by government as a % of GDP from the existing 0.9 % to 2%.	
12)	Increase share of central grants to constitute at least 25 %of total health spending.	2010
13)	Further increase to 8% of the total budget	2010
	Eliminate lymphatic Filariasis.	2015

National Health Policy 2017

The Union Cabinet approved National Health Policy 2017, proposing to provide *"Assured Health services to all"*. For the first time, the Government set a time-bound target with a limited deadline to strengthen the healthcare system in India. The previous policies were **cure -centric** and a new one is preventive and **patient-centric** with quality-driven. Earlier policy focused on communicable diseases but over the last 10-15 years the focus has been shifted towards non-communicable diseases which caused the majority of deaths.NHP, 2017 promises **'assured health care for all at affordable cost'** and changes the discourse of **Health for all** to **'Health in all'.**

Goals of the Policy: The policy aims:

- To attain the **highest possible level of health and wellbeing for all** ages, through a preventive and promotive health care orientation.

- To provide **universal access to good quality health care** services without anyone having to face financial burden. This would be achieved through increasing access, lowering the cost, and improving the quality of health care delivery.

Objective: The primary objective of the National Health Policy, 2017 is:

- **To strengthen the common man's interest in the public health care system** by making it patient-centric, efficient, effective, and affordable, with a comprehensive (that includes everything) package of services and products that meet the immediate health care needs of most people.

- To inform, clarify, strengthen and prioritize the role of the Government in shaping the health system in all its dimensions.

Key features of NHP 2017:

- **Assurance-Based Approach**: Policy advocates progressively incremental Assurance based Approach with a focus on preventive and promotive healthcare.

- The Indian government has declared to increase **expenditure on healthcare to 2.5%** of GDP which is currently 1.5 %. The rise in expenditure will be achieved phase-wise by 2025.

- The government will provide **free medication & diagnosis tests** in all public hospitals to make sure every citizen of the country accesses all health facilities irrespective of financial status.

- **Health Card linked to health facilities**– Government will provide health cards to each patient to maintain the patient's history digitally.

- Previously the role of the primary health centers was immunization & check-ups. The new policy includes the screening of non-communicable diseases also.

- **Up-gradation of district hospitals** with new framework implementation.

- Good health &Yoga would be introduced widely in workplaces and schools.

- **Patient-Centric Approach**: The policy recommends setting up a separate, empowered medical tribunal for a speedy resolution to address disputes

/complaints regarding standards of care, services price, negligence, and unfair practices.

➢ **Micronutrient Deficiency:** Focus on reducing micronutrient malnourishment.

➢ **Quality of Care**: Public hospitals and facilities would undergo periodic measurements and certification of the level of quality.

➢ **Make in India Initiative:** Policy advocates the need to enhance local manufacturing of customized medicines and infrastructure.

➢ **Application of Digital Health:** Policy emphasizes the use of digital tools for improving the efficiency and outcome of the healthcare system.

➢ **Private Sector engagement for strategic purchase** for critical gap filling and the achievement of health goals.

➢ To get services situations, the policy has provision to provide emergency services free of cost in all care levels in public hospitals for that it aims to ensure the availability of two beds per 1,000 population to enable access within a golden hour [the first hour after traumatic injury, when the victim is most likely to benefit from emergency treatment].

Specific Quantifiable Goals: NHP 2017 also sets **specific measurable, time-bound goals in three core areas** to track the attainment of policy objectives:

a) Health Status and Program impact,

b) Health Systems Performance,

c) Health Systems Strengthening.

Table 1.3 List of key quantitative indicators

		Health Status and Programme Impact
1	**Life Expectancy and healthy life**	Increase Life Expectancy at birth from 67.5 to 70 by 2025.
		Establish regular tracking of the Disability Adjusted Life Years (DALY) Index as a measure of the burden of disease and its trends by major categories by 2022.
		Reduction of Total Fertility Rate (TFR) to 2.1 at national and sub-national levels by 2025. In FY 2016, India had a TFR of 2.3 birth per woman.
2	**Mortality by Age and/ or cause**	Reduce Under Five Mortality to 23 by 2025 and **Maternal Mortality Ratio** MMR from current levels 167 to 100 by 2020
		Reduce infant mortality rate to 28 by 2019, the IMR was 34 per 1000 live births in 2015.
		Reduce neonatal mortality to 16 and stillbirth rate to "single digit" by 2025

Table 1.3 *contd…*

3	Reduction of disease prevalence/ incidence	Achieve the global target of 2020 which is also termed as a target of 90:90:90, for HIV/AIDS i.e.90% of all people living with HIV know their HIV status, –90% of all people diagnosed with HIV infection receive sustained antiretroviral therapy and 90% of all people receiving antiretroviral therapy will have viral suppression.
		Achieve and maintain elimination status of Leprosy by 2018, Kala-Azar by 2017, and Lymphatic Filariasis in endemic pockets by 2017.
		To achieve and maintain a cure rate of >85% in new sputum-positive patients for TB and reduce the incidence of new cases, to reach elimination status by 2025.
		To reduce the prevalence of blindness to 0.25/1000 by 2025 and the disease burden by one-third from current levels.
		To reduce premature mortality from cardiovascular diseases, cancer, diabetes, or chronic respiratory diseases by 25% by 2025.
Health Systems Performance		
1	Coverage of Health Services	Increase utilization of public health facilities by 50% from current levels by **2025.**
		Antenatal care coverage to be sustained above 90% and skilled attendance at birth above 90% by **2025.**
		More than 90% of newborns are fully immunized by one year of age by **2025.**
		Meet the need for family planning above 90% at the national and sub-national levels by **2025.**
		80% of known hypertensive and diabetic individuals at the household level maintained, controlled disease status" by **2025**
2	Cross-Sectoral goals related to health	The relative reduction in the prevalence of current tobacco use by 15% by 2020 and 30% by 2025.
		Reduction of 40% in the prevalence of stunting of under-five children by 2025.
		Access to safe water and sanitation to all by 2020 (Swachh Bharat Mission)
		Reduction of occupational injury by half from current levels of 334 per lakh agricultural workers by 2020.
		National/ State level tracking of selected health behavior.
Health Systems strengthening		
1	Health finance	Increase health expenditure by Government as a percentage of GDP from the existing 1.15% to 2.5 % by 2025.
		Increase State sector health spending to > 8% of their budget by 2020.

Table 1.3 *contd…*

		Decrease in the proportion of households facing catastrophic health expenditure from the current levels by 25%, by 2025.
2	**Health Infrastructure and Human Resource**	Ensure availability of paramedics and doctors as per the Indian Public Health Standard (IPHS) norm in high-priority districts by 2020.
		Increase community health volunteers to population ratio as per IPHS norm, in high-priority districts by **2025.**
		Establish primary and secondary care facilities as per norms in high-priority districts (population as well as time to reach norms) by **2025.**
3	**Health Management Information**	Ensure district-level electronic database of information on health system components by 2020.
		Strengthen the health surveillance system and establish registries for diseases of public health importance by 2020.
		Establish federated integrated health information architecture, Health Information Exchanges, and National Health Information Network by 2025.
Health Status and Programme Impact		
1	**Life Expectancy and healthy life**	Increase Life Expectancy at birth from 67.5 to 70 by 2025.
		Establish regular tracking of the disability Adjusted Life Years (DALY) Index as a measure of the burden of disease and its trends by major categories by 2022.
		Reduction of Total Fertility Rate (TFR) to 2.1 at national and sub-national levels by 2025. In FY 2016, India had TFR of 2.3 birth per woman.
2	**Mortality by Age and/ or cause**	Reduce Under Five Mortality to 23 by 2025 and Maternal Mortality Ratio MMR from current levels 167 to 100 by 2020
		Reduce infant mortality rate to 28 by 2019, the IMR was 34 per 1000 live births in 2015.
		Reduce neonatal mortality to 16 and stillbirth rate to "single-digit" by 2025
3	**Reduction of disease prevalence/ incidence**	Achieve the global target of 2020 which is also termed as the target of 90:90:90, for HIV/AIDS i.e,90% of all people living with HIV know their HIV status, –90% of all people diagnosed with HIV infection receive sustained antiretroviral therapy and 90% of all people receiving antiretroviral therapy will have viral suppression.
		Achieve and maintain elimination status of Leprosy by 2018, Kala-Azar by 2017, and Lymphatic Filariasis in endemic pockets by 2017.
		To achieve and maintain a cure rate of >85% in new sputum-positive patients for TB and reduce the incidence of new cases, to reach elimination status by 2025.

Table 1.3 *contd…*

		To reduce the prevalence of blindness to 0.25/1000 by 2025 and the disease burden by one-third from current levels.
		To reduce premature mortality from cardiovascular diseases, cancer, diabetes, or chronic respiratory diseases by 25% by 2025.
Health Systems Performance		
1	**Coverage of Health Services**	Increase utilization of public health facilities by 50% from current levels by **2025.**
		Antenatal care coverage to be sustained above 90% and skilled attendance at birth above 90% by **2025.**
		More than 90% of newborns are fully immunized by one year of age by **2025.**
		Meet the need for family planning above 90% at the national sub-national level by **2025.**
		80% of known hypertensive and diabetic individuals at the household level maintained, controlled disease status" by **2025**
2	**Cross-Sectoral goals related to health**	The relative reduction in the prevalence of current tobacco useby 15% by 2020 and 30% by 2025.
		Reduction of 40% in the prevalence of stunting of under-five children by 2025.
		Access to safe water and sanitation to all by 2020 (Swachh Bharat Mission)
		Reduction of occupational injury by half from current levels of 334 per lakh agricultural workers by 2020.
		National/ State level tracking of selected health behaviour.
Health Systems strengthening		
1	**Health finance**	Increase health expenditure by Government as a percentage of GDP from the existing 1.15% to 2.5 % by 2025.
		Increase state sector health spending to > 8% of their budget by 2020.
		Decrease in the proportion of households facing catastrophic health expenditure from the current levels by 25%, by 2025.
2	**Health Infrastructure and Human Resource**	Ensure availability of paramedics and doctors as per the Indian Public Health Standard (IPHS) norm in high-priority districts by 2020.
		Increase community health volunteers to population ratio as per IPHS norm, in high-priority districts by **2025.**

Table 1.3 *contd…*

		Establish primary and secondary care facilities as per norms in high-priority districts (population as well as time to reach norms) by **2025.**
3	**Health Management Information**	Ensure district-level electronic database of information on health system components by 2020.
		Strengthen the health surveillance system and establish registries for diseases of public health importance by 2020.
		Establish federated integrated health information architecture, Health Information Exchanges, and National Health Information Network by 2025.

Figure 1.4 Various National Health Policies

New reform policy has risen in expenditure limits with schemes like free medication & emergency services. Following are the few challenges India is facing in achieving the goals of NHP 2017:

- 100 percent utilization of allocated amount in targeted care service not achieved.
- Lack of resources in regulatory authority (FDA/NAPPA/CDSCO) & in all levels of care services.
- Lack of infrastructure available in the rural area.

- Lack of right intention & willingness to provide service, not the product.
- Due to the bad quality of services people are shifting towards private services which leads to a financial burden on them.
- Unavailability of highly integrated systems/devices in public hospitals.
- With loose control of the government over the whole healthcare system except (DCO),drug manufacturers are free to set drug prices.
- Lack of strict guidelines pharma industry to maintain the high-quality of medicines (violation of GMP guidelines).

Other than the NHPs, many other policies were announced from time to time that are closely linked with improving the health status of people. Some of such National Policies are listed in the table.

Table 1.4 National health policies/other related policies for the promotion of health

YEAR	NAME OF POLICY
1983	**National Health Policy**
1992	National AIDS Control and Prevention Policy
1993	National Nutrition Policy
1999	National Policy on Older Persons
2000	National Population Policy
2001	National Policy for Empowerment of Women
2002	National Blood Policy
2002	National Policy on Indian System of Medicine and Homeopathy
2002	**National Health Policy**
2003	National Policy for Access to Plasma-derived Medicinal Products from Human Plasma for Clinical/Therapeutic use
2003	National charter for children
2005	National Rural Health Mission
2006	National Environment Policy
2009	Right of children to Free and Compulsory Education Bill (education to children aged between 6 and 14 years)
2012	National Pharmaceutical Pricing Policy
2012	National Water Policy
2013	National Policy for Children
2015	National Youth Policy
2017	**National Health Policy**

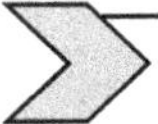

1.5   Public and Private Healthcare Systems in India

The terms health system and healthcare system are often used interchangeably but there is quite a big difference between these.

➤ Health care systems are limited to personal healthcare services, such as curative services.

➤ Health systems encompass wider dimensions of health, such as social and economic determinants of health.

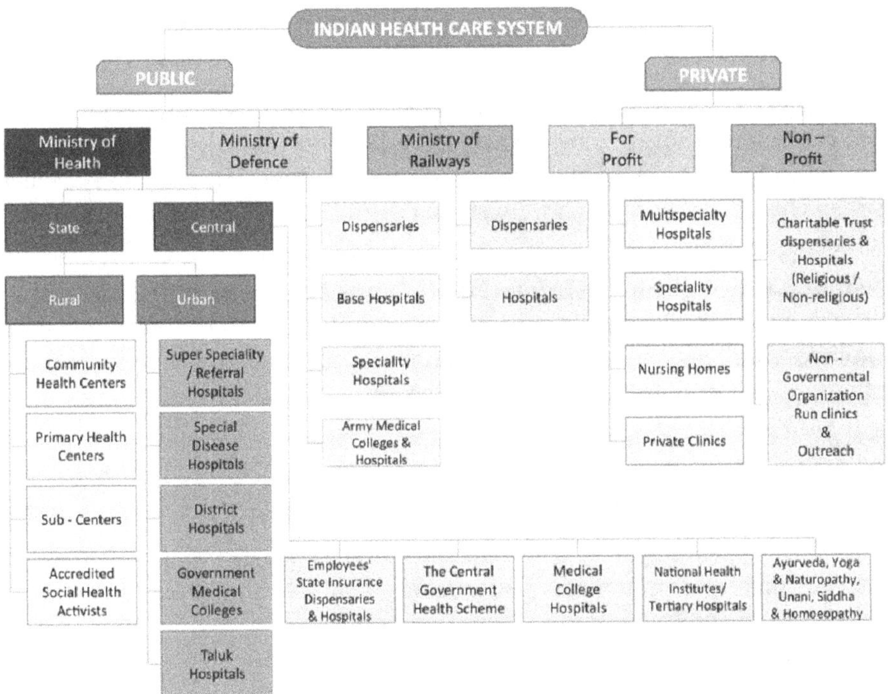

Figure 1.5 Indian healthcare system

Indian Health care Systems: Indian healthcare system is divided into two sectors: Public and private.

Public Sector Healthcare: The public healthcare industry (operated by the Indian government) is responsible for providing health services and treatments to all people. This sector includes super-specialty hospitals equipped with medicines and instruments, which are majorly located in tier I and tier-II cities. Additionally, district- and taluka-level hospitals provide healthcare services to the people. Primary healthcare centers and village hospitals with low costs are available, which provide affordable services to the people.

Private Sector Healthcare: This has a similar structure and provides amenities and services to the middle-class and upper-class people in India.

The overall cost of healthcare services included in the private sector is higher than that in the public sector. Technological interventions are also more diverse in the private sector than in the public sector. The figure illustrates the detailed structure of the Indian healthcare system.

Non-profit hospitals: Non-profit hospitals are community hospitals and their main goal is to provide free–of–cost services to the community. The funds to run such hospitals are raised from the donations and offerings given by the people.

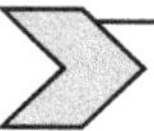

1.6   National Health Mission

The National Health Mission was launched by the Indian government in 2013 and is being implemented by the Ministry of Family and Health Welfare. The project merged two previous missions, National Rural Health, and National Urban Health, both of which were started in 2005 with the goal of addressing India's malnutrition crisis.

National Rural Health Mission (NRHM) was launched on April 12, 2005, to address the health needs of the underserved rural population especially women, children, and vulnerable sections of the society, and to provide affordable, accessible, and quality healthcare.

National Urban Health Mission (NUUM): NUHM aims to satisfy the health care needs of the urban population, with a particular focus on the urban poor, by making critical primary health care services available to them and lowering their out-of-pocket treatment costs.

The main programmatic components include the strengthening of healthcare in rural and urban areas, Reproductive-Maternal-Neonatal-Child and Adolescent health (RMNCH+A)

In March 2018, it was extended again with a wider focus on establishing a fully functional, community-owned, decentralized health delivery system with inter-sectoral convergence at all levels, to ensure simultaneous action on a wide range of determinants of health such as education, clean water, sanitation, nutrition, and gender equality

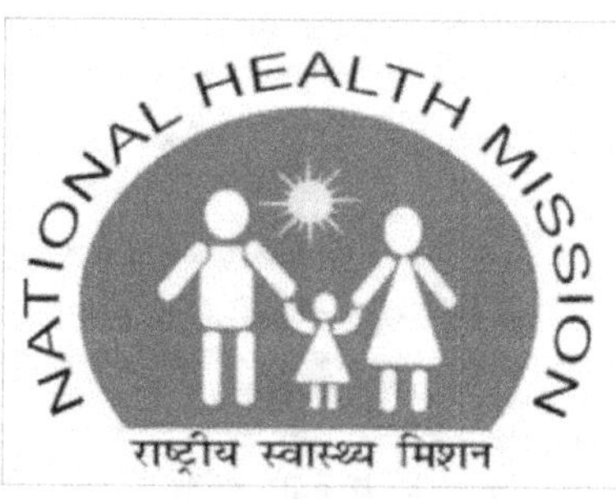

Objective: The overall objective of the National Health Mission is to ensure that everyone gets easy access to high- quality affordable health care services, accountable and responsive to people's needs

Goals of the National Health Mission

National Health Mission is basically a conglomerate of all existing health schemes of the country. The broad measurable objectives of this mission in totality are as follows:

➤ Reducing MMR to 1/1000 live births

➤ Reducing IMR to 25/1000 live births

➤ Reducing TFR (Total Fertility Rate) to 2.1

➤ Prevention of anaemia in women aged 15-49 years

➤ Prevent and reduce mortality & morbidity from communicable, non-communicable

➤ Injuries and emerging diseases

➤ Reduce household out-of-pocket expenditure on total health care expenditure

➤ Reduce annual incidence and mortality from Tuberculosis by half

➤ Reduce the prevalence of Leprosy to <1/10000 population and incidence to zero in all districts

➤ Annual Malaria Incidence to be <1/1000

➤ Less than 1 percent microfilaria prevalence in all districts

➤ Kala-azar elimination by 2015, <1 case per 10000 population in all blocks

Components of NHM

1. National Rural Health Mission (now called NRHM-RCH Flexipool)
2. National Urban Health Mission Flexipool for populations above 50000
3. Flexible pool for Communicable disease
4. Flexible pool for Non-communicablediseases including Injury and Trauma
5. Infrastructure Maintenance
6. Family Welfare Central Sector component.

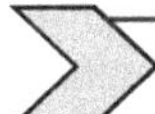 **1.7   Millennium Development Goals (MDG's)**

The WHO's Vision of Health for All by 2000 AD failed due to a lack of defined targets and indicators, poor planning, lack of expert help, insufficient budgets, and poor commitment towards its implementation.

The UN General Assembly (UNGA) convened the Millennium Summit in September 2000, where all 189 Member States adopted the Millennium Declaration, a statement of values, principles, and objectives for the twenty-first century. The member nations pledged to free people from extreme poverty and hunger, disease, illiteracy, environmental degradation, and discrimination against women. This pledge became the eight Millennium Development Goals to be achieved by 2015. In September 2010, the world recommitted itself to accelerate progress towards these goals.

The **Eight Millennium Development Goals** are:

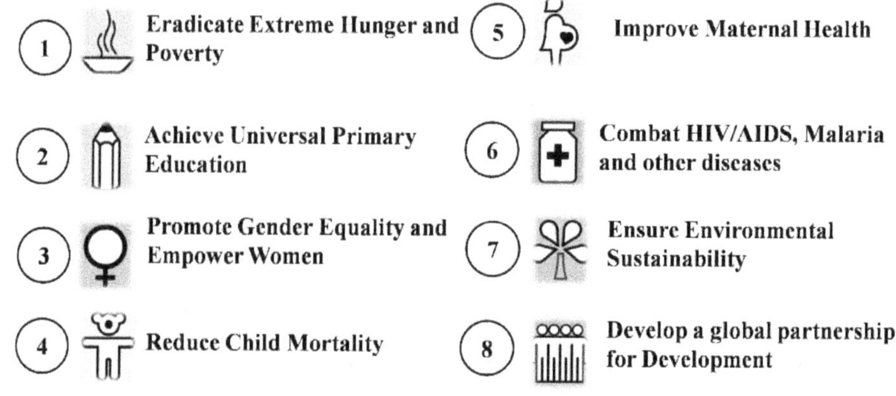

Figure 1.6 Millenium Development Goals

Eighteen (18) targets were set as quantitative markers for attaining the goals. The United Nations Development Group (UNDG) in 2003 provided a framework of 53 indicators which were categorized according to targets, for measuring the progress towards individual targets India's MDG framework was based on the 2003 framework and included **8 goals, 12 targets relevant to India, and 35 indicators.**

In brief, globally, the MDGs helped lift **more than 1 billion people out of extreme poverty,** made plans against hunger, **improved school enrollment rates,** and **protected the planet.** The MDG process **created new partnerships, improved public opinion about such global development processes,** and demonstrated the value of setting ambitious goals.

India's Progress towards achieving the Millenium Development Goals

India's progress towards achieving the Millennium Development Goals

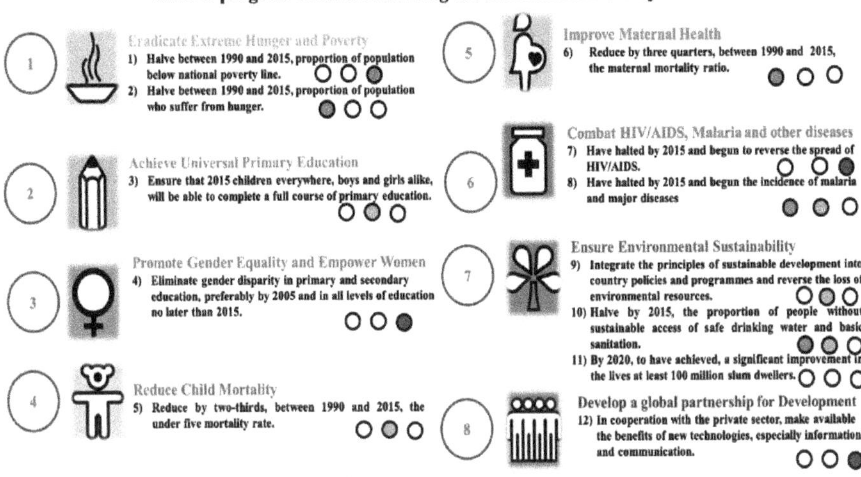

Figure 1.7 India's Progress in achieving MDG

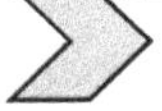

1.8 Sustainable Development Goals

It is our responsibility to build a bright and sustainable future for our children and our planet.

Sustainable development is the development that meets the needs of the present without disturbing future generations to meet their own needs. It is based on the three pillars of sustainability economic, environmental and social sustainability.

End of MDGs: During 15 years of MDGs, progress was observed in several important areas. The achievements of MDGs provided us with valuable lessons and experience to begin work on new goals. The term of MDGs was to end on December 31, 2015, but the world was still plagued with global issues such as poverty, inequality, environmental degradation, human violence, and abuse.

United Nations Sustainable Development Summit: In September 2015, The UN Sustainable Development Summit (meeting) was convened, and approximately 193 Member States participated. The United Nations General Assembly (UNGA) set up a collection of **17 goals** known as the **sustainable development goals or** simply **'Global Goals'.** All the participating member states agreed to adopt *"Transforming our World: The 2030 Agenda for Sustainable Development."*

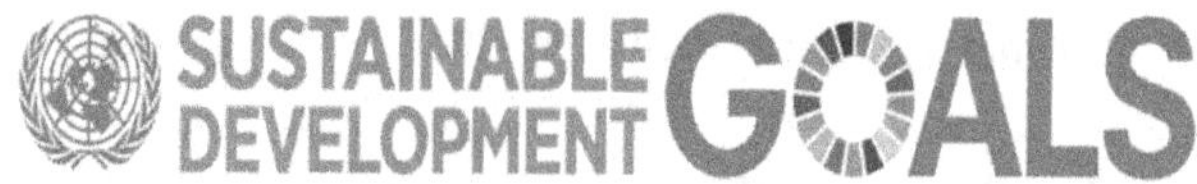

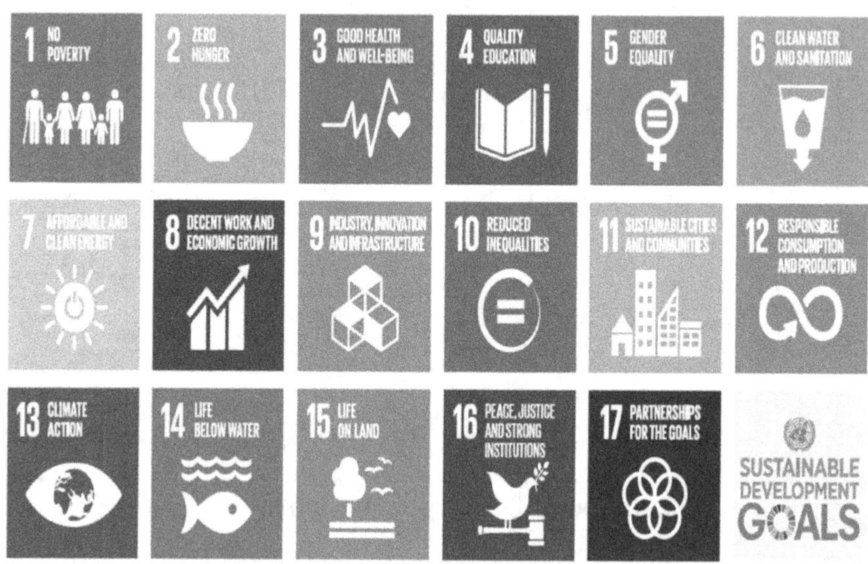

Figure 1.8 Sustainable Development Goals

Start of SDGs: It was termed as **2030 Agenda for Sustainable Development** and later its name was shortened to **2030 AGENDA.** This Agenda proposed a roadmap for ending global poverty, building a life of dignity, and pledging *to leave no one behind.* It came into force on **1st January 2016 and will work until 2030.**

Execution of SDGs: The member countries are expected to form their own sustainable development policies plans and programs. They would be responsible for implementing these policies in order to achieve the defined goals and targets. These **17 international** Sustainable Development Goals are a 'to-do list for the planet that will transform the world' achieving these goals involves making very big fundamental changes in how we live on Earth this is called transformation Through these goals we need to transform the way we stay on this earth.

The main focus of MDGs was on developing countries but the Sustainable Development Goals are universal, **integrated and interconnected.**

➢ **Universality** means that these goals apply to every nation, every sector, every city, every business school, and organization.
➢ All the goals are **integrated and interconnected** as we cannot aim to achieve just one goal we must achieve them all this is called integration.

The SDGs cover a broad range of sustainability issues that encompass economic, social, and environmental dimensions. These include poverty, hunger, health, education, climate change, gender equality, water supply, sanitation, energy, urbanization, environment, and social justice.

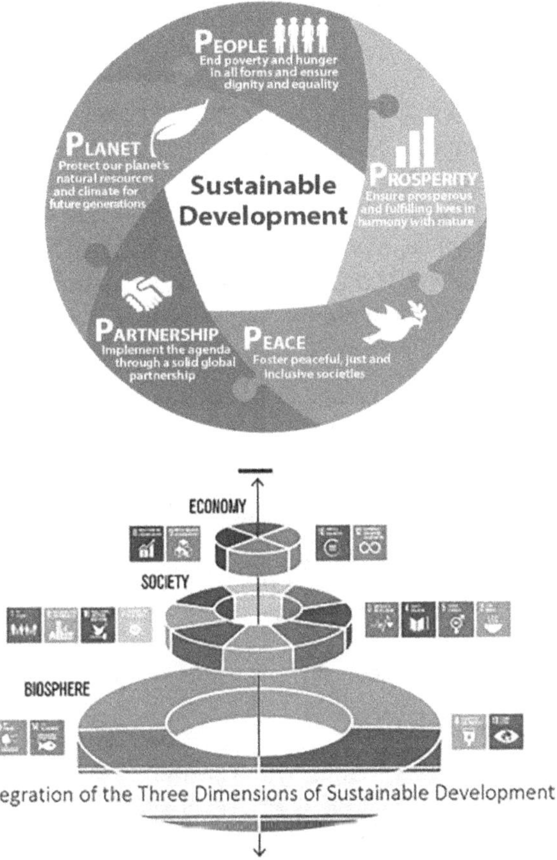

Figure 1.9 Five dimensions to achieve Sustainable Development

The 2030 Agenda is based on **five dimensions,** also known as the 5Ps:

➢ **People**: To **end poverty and hunger**, in all their forms and dimensions, and to ensure that all human beings can fulfill their potential in dignity and equality and a healthy environment.

➢ **Planet:** To protect the planet from degradation through **sustainable consumption and production, sustainably managing its natural resources,** and taking urgent action on climate change.

➢ **Prosperity:** To ensure that all human beings can enjoy prosperous and fulfilling lives and that **economic, social, and technological progress** occurs in harmony with nature.

➢ **Peace:** To foster **peaceful, just, and inclusive societies** which are free from fear and violence.

➢ **Partnership:** To mobilize the means required to implement the 2030 Agenda through **apartnershipbased on a spirit of solidarity** and focused, in particular, on the needs of the most vulnerable.

SDGS AND INDIA

To achieve the SDGs, the Indian Government is working on the proposed framework to **leave no one behind.** The motto of **Sabka Saath Sabka Vikas** and the flagship programs like **Swachh Bharat Mission, Beti Bachao Beti Padhao, Pradhan mantra Aawas Yojana, Pradhan Mantri Jan Dhan Yojana, etc** highlight the Government's commitment to the development that it reaches to all its citizens. The focus is also on connecting villages with roads, health programs, expansion of digital connectivity, Universal health coverage, sanitation, and housing for all.

The SDG Index is an assessment of each country's overall performance on the 17 SDGs, giving equal weight to each Goal. The score signifies a country's position between the worst possible outcome (0) and the best, or target outcome (100). **The report on sustainable development goals in 2021** reported India in a very comfortable position.

India is at 120th rank with an SDG index of 60.1 as compared to Finland which ranks first with an SDG index of 85.9.

Table 1.5 The 17 Sustainable Development Goals: Agenda 2030

SDG Goal	Key features
1 NO POVERTY **To end poverty in all its forms everywhere**	The objective of **SDG 1** is to ensure that the entire population especially the poorest and most vulnerable have equal rights to economic resources, access to basic services, property and land control, natural resources and new technologies.
2 ZERO HUNGER **To end global hunger and malnutrition**	**Goal 2** seeks sustainable solutions to end hunger in all its forms by 2030 and to achieve food security. The aim is to ensure that everyone everywhere has enough good-quality food to lead a healthy life. Achieving this Goal will require better access to food and the widespread promotion of sustainable agriculture.

Table 1.5 *contd...*

SDG Goal	Key features
To ensure healthy lives and promote well-being for all at all ages	Based on the interdependence of health and development, **SDG 3** aspires to ensure health and well-being for all, with a bold commitment to end the epidemics of AIDS, tuberculosis, malaria and other communicable diseases by 2030. It also aims to achieve universal health coverage, and provide access to safe and effective medicines and vaccines for all.
To ensure inclusive and equitable quality education and promote lifelong learning opportunities for all	Education is one of the most powerful and proven vehicles for sustainable development. **SDG 4** ensures that all girls and boys complete free primary and secondary schooling by 2030. It also aims to provide equal access to affordable vocational training, and to eliminate gender and wealth disparities with the aim of achieving universal access to a quality higher education.
To Achieve gender equality and empower all women and girls	**The women and girls being half of the world's population and equality is their fundamental right.** Empowered women and girls contribute to the health and productivity of their families, communities, and countries, **Goal 5** aims to eliminate all forms of discrimination and violence against women in the public and private spheres and to undertake reforms to give women equal rights to economic resources and access to ownership of property.
To ensure availability and sustainable management of water and sanitation for all.	Availability and access to water, sanitation and hygiene (WASH) services is fundamental for fighting against the diseases and preserving the health and well-being of millions. **SDG 6 focuses** on ensuring a clean and stable water supply and effective water sanitation for all people by the year 2030.

Table 1.5 *contd…*

SDG Goal	Key features
To ensure universal access to affordable, reliable and modern energy services	Expanding infrastructure and upgrading technology to provide clean and more efficient energy in all countries will encourage growth and help the environment. Investing in solar, wind and thermal power, improving energy productivity, and ensuring energy for all is vital if we are to achieve **SDG 7** by 2030.
To promote inclusive and sustainable economic growth, employment and decent work for all.	Sustained and inclusive economic growth can drive progress, create decent jobs for all and improve living standards. **SDG 8 aims** to achieve full and productive employment and decent work for all women and men, including for young people and persons with disabilities, and equal pay for work of equal value by 2030.
To build resilient infrastructure, promote inclusive and sustainable industrialization and foster innovation.	**SDG 9** encompasses three important aspects of sustainabledevelopment: infrastructure,industrialization,andinnovation. To meet future challenges, our industries and infrastructure must be upgraded with an emphasis on greater adoption of clean and environmentally sound technologies and industrial processes and increased resource-use efficiency.
To reduce inequality within and among countries.	This SDG calls for reducing inequalities in income as well as those based on age, sex, disability, race, ethnicity, origin, religion, or economic or other status within a country. Reducing inequality requires **transformative change**. Greater efforts are needed to eradicate extreme poverty and hunger, and invest more in health, education, social protection, and decent jobs especially for young people, migrants and refugees and other vulnerable communities.

Table 1.5 *contd...*

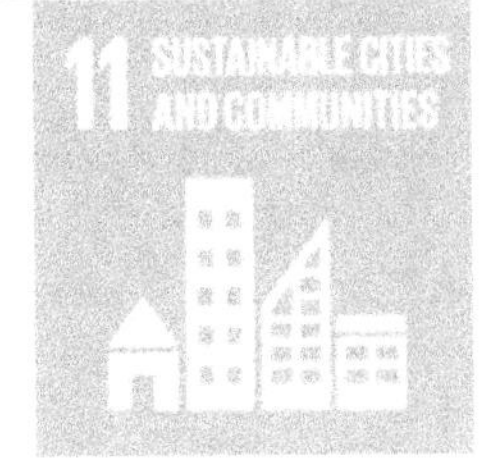 To Make cities inclusive, safe, resilient and sustainable	According To SDG 11 we need to renew and plan cities and other human settlements in a way that offers opportunities for all, with access to basic services, energy, housing, transportation and green public spaces, while reducing resource use and environmental impact.
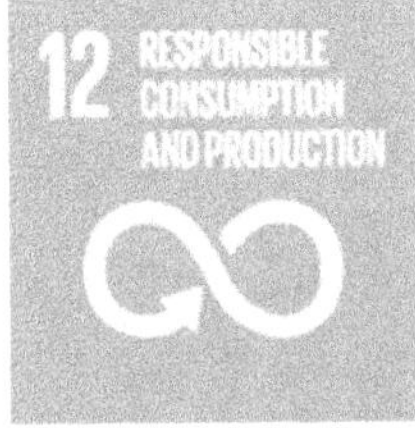 **To ensure sustainable Consumption and production patterns;**	SDG 12 is meant to ensure good use of resources, improving energy efficiency, sustainable infrastructure, and providing access to basic services, green and decent jobs and ensuring a better quality of life for all. Sustainable consumption and production aims at "doing more and better with less," **increasing net welfare gains from economic activities by reducing resource use, degradation, and pollution**, while increasing the quality of life.
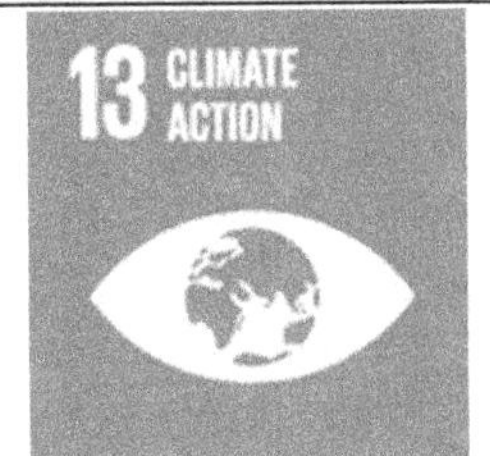 take urgent action to combat climate change and its effects	**The Earth's weather patterns are changing** and human activity is largely responsible for this climate change has a negative impact on the environment, the economy, human well-being and communities and, if we do not act fast, the consequences will be devastating for life and for the development of our planet.
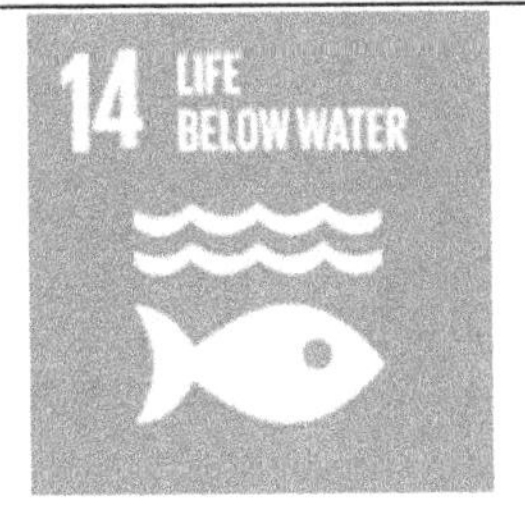 Conserve and sustainably use the oceans, seas and marine resources	The world's oceans – their temperature, chemistry, currents and life – drive global systems that make the Earth habitable for humankind. The **SDG 14** aims to sustainably manage and protect marine and coastal ecosystems from land-based pollution, as well as address the impacts of ocean acidification. An emphasis on conservation and the sustainable use of ocean-based resources will also help in the prevention of related challenges.

Table 1.5 *contd…*

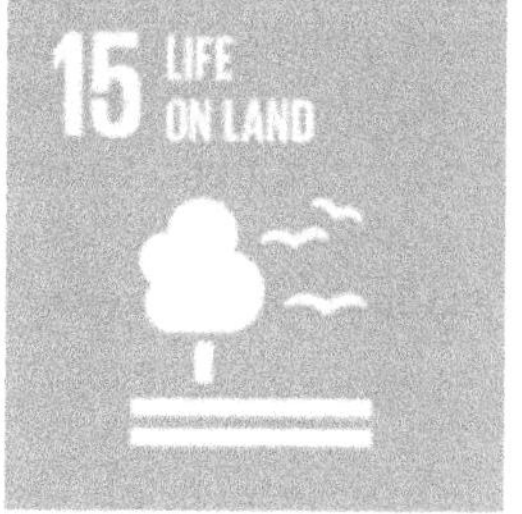 **manage forests, combat desertification, halt and reverse land degradation and halt biodiversity loss".**	**SDG 15** aims to protect, restore and promote the sustainable use of terrestrial ecosystems by halting deforestation to protect natural habitats and threatened species. If SDG 15 is carried out, the world's forests, mountains, drylands, and wetlands will be conserved and restored by 2030.
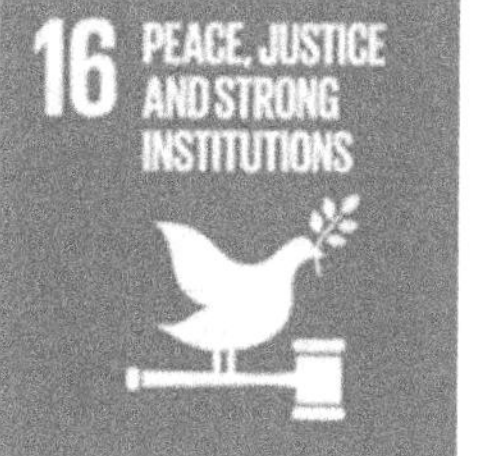 **To promote just, peaceful and inclusive societies.**	SDG 16 aims to promote peaceful and inclusive societies for sustainable development and to provide access to justice for all and build effective, accountable and inclusive institutions at all levels.
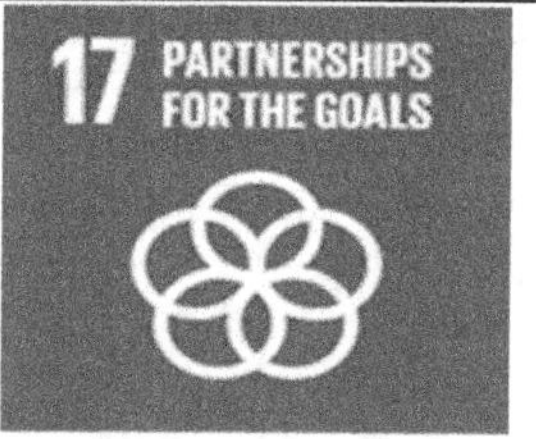 **To revitalize the Global Partnership for Sustainable Development**	**SDG 17** is a vision for improved and more equitable trade, as well as coordinated investment initiatives to promote sustainable development across borders. Assist developing countries in attaining long-term debt sustainability through coordinated policies aimed at fostering debt financing, debt relief, and debt restructuring by 2030.

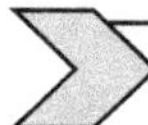 **1.9   FIP Development Goals**

International Pharmaceutical Federation (FIP): The FIP is the global federation of national associations of pharmacists and pharmaceutical scientists, representing three million pharmacists and scientists through its 127 Member Organisations.

Its mission is *"to improve global health by advancing pharmacy practice and science to enable better discovery, development, access to and safe use of appropriate, cost-effective, quality medicines worldwide."*

Need for FIP Development Goals: The WHO Global Strategy for *Human Resources for Health: Workforce* **2030**focused on "No health without a workforce". Building on this statement, FIP framed its strategic plan to map and meet national and global health challenges through workforce development and transformation. FIP believes that we can have no pharmaceutical care without a pharmaceutical workforce, and without a scientific foundation. The pharmaceutical workforce is a unique profession with diverse expertise covering science, practice and education.

In September 2020, the **FIP published a set of 21 Development Goals (DGs)** that bring together the workforce and education, practice, and science in a transformative framework, defining an improved and more advanced pharmacy profession for the next decade. The FIP DGs form a foundation for systematic action to meet national, regional, and global healthcare needs.

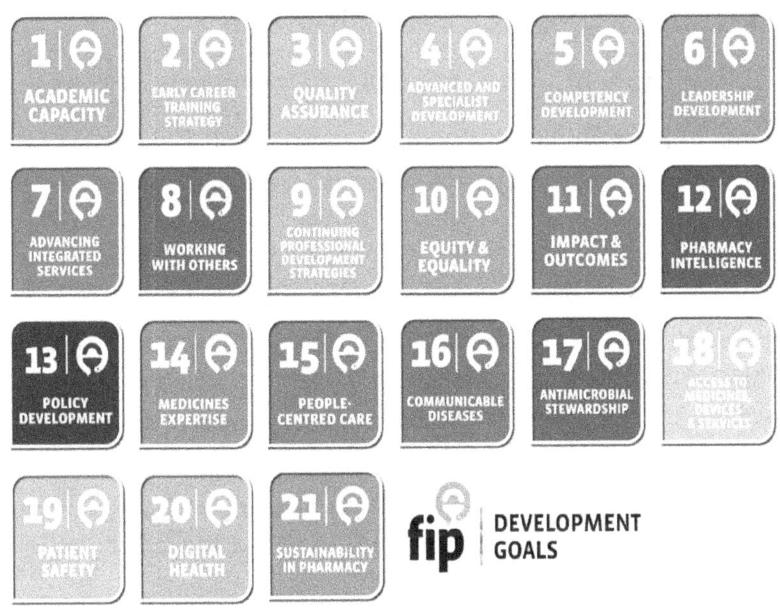

Figure 1.10 FIP Development Goals

Objectives of FIP DGs

➢ The FIP Development Goals are a major global initiative for pharmacy and are a key resource for **transforming the pharmacy profession over the next decade** globally, regionally, and nationally.

➢ Goals provide the global pharmacy with a logical next step **to link the pharmaceutical workforce with pharmaceutical healthcare provision and the pharmaceutical services we deliver.**

➢ Goals necessitate **bringing science, practice, workforce, and education together** through the 21 Development Goals to provide us with a roadmap and priorities for the next decade.

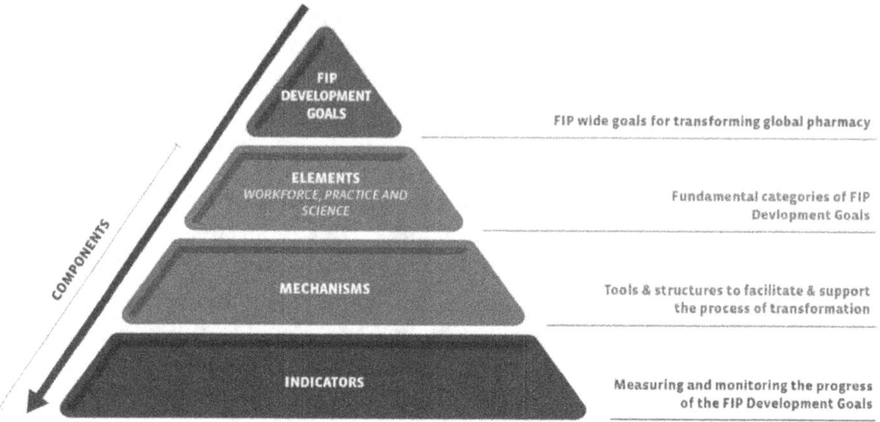

Figure 1.11 Key categories of FIP Development Goals

Execution of FIP DGs: It is believed that for all members there should be one common transformative framework to bring science, practice, and workforce & education together. The concept helped in setting the "One FIP" Development Goals (common goals) for the development of the pharmacy profession in the next decade.

Each of the FIP DGs is composed of 3 Elements for Practice, Science, and Workforce that all form fundamental categories of the Goals. Alongside each Element is a set of mechanisms that form tools and structures to facilitate and support the process of transformation.

Significance of FIP Goals: The 21 DGs are accompanied by a growing set of FIP global tools, structures, indicators, and programs to facilitate and support the process of transformation.

➢ The FIP DGs serve as a systematic framework for needs assessment and mapping priorities.

➢ FIP serves to facilitate monitoring, a dashboard, and a system of sharing best practice development, globally and regionally, with evidence generated and displayed through the FIP Global Pharmaceutical Observatory and the FIP Atlas.

➢ The FIP platform provides opportunities for members and partners to share and support developments nationally, regionally, and globally through partnerships.

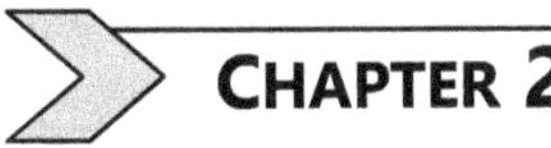

CHAPTER 2

Role of Pharmacist in Preventive Health Care

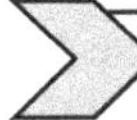

2.1 Demography and Family Planning

The population of any country is in a continuous state of change both in terms of its size and characteristics. Fertility is one of the main components of population growth. High fertility results in rapid population growth. To determine if fertility is declining, increasing, or remaining the same, the assessments are made through demographic analysis. National and State level projections help the policymakers and program implementers across the government ministries to assess the population size, and future projections to identify the community's unmet needs. The Sustainable Development Goals (SDGs) call on countries to ensure universal access to sexual and reproductive health-care services, including family planning, information and education, and the integration of reproductive health into national strategies and programs by 2030.

LEARNING OBJECTIVES

- Demography and Family Planning
- Mother and child health, the importance of breastfeeding, ill effects of infant milk substitutes and bottle feeding
- Overview of Vaccines, types of immunity, and immunization
- Effect of Environment on Health – water pollution, the importance of safe drinking water, waterborne diseases, air pollution, noise pollution, sewage, and solid waste disposal, occupational illnesses, Environmental pollution due to pharmaceuticals
- Psychosocial Pharmacy: Drugs of misuse and abuse – psychotropics, narcotics, alcohol, tobacco products. Social Impact of these habits on social health and productivity and suicidal behaviors

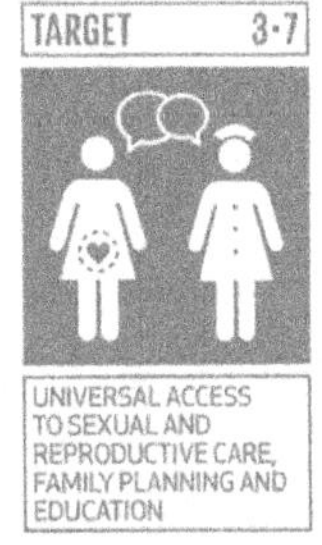

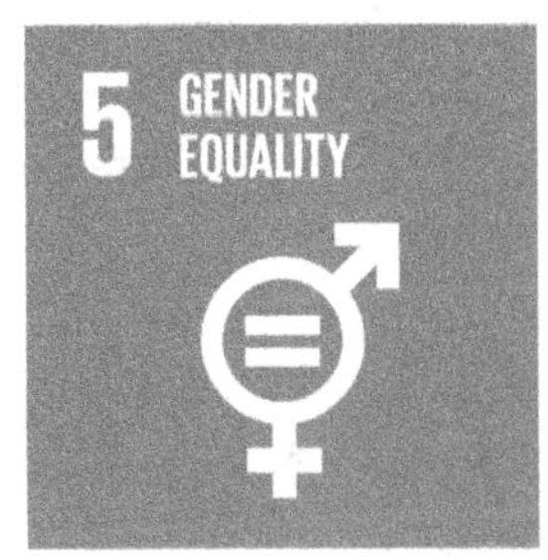

India is working tirelessly to improve health and reduce fertility in order to achieve SDG 3.

Demography

The term is of Greek origin and is composed of the two words, demos (people) and graphein (describe). *Demography* is the systematic study of the human population with respect to size, composition, distribution, and changes in the population that occur over time.

Populations are never static; the number of people in a given area can grow or decline as a result of the number of births that take place, the number of deaths that occur, and/or the number of people moving in or out of a locale. The interplay of three demographic processes is responsible for the growth/decline in population, these are:

1. **Fertility:** Fertility is a demographic indicator that refers to a population's actual reproduction performance based on the number of live births that occur. It shows the number of children who were born alive. Childbearing is influenced by a variety of factors, including societal circumstances such as culture, tradition, education, and a society's or community's general degree of development. In addition, the age at which a couple enters a relationship and the availability of contraception are two important factors of fertility.

2. **Mortality:** Death of an individual or the number of deaths that occur in a population.

3. **Migration:** The movement of people into or out of a specific geographic area. Migration can drastically change the size and composition of a population in a brief period of time, especially in small geographic locations.

Stages of Demography: Demography in any country broadly moves through five stages

➤ In the first stage, a country experiences high birth rates and death rates leading to a stagnant population with low life expectancy.

➤ Falling crude death rates (CDR) and high crude birth rates (CBR) indicate the start of the **second phase** of demographic transition.
An alarming expansion of the population in the form of children in the age group of 0-14 years is observed.

➤ With increased education, fertility rates gradually fall, and in the third stage, the population of adults who are economically active increases in a nation.

➤ In the Fourth stage, the population stabilizes with the birth and death rates generally equalizing, while the average life expectancy (age) of the population gradually increases.

➤ In the final fifth phase of demographic transition the death rates exceed birth rates and it manifests as a decline in population growth.

Table 2.1 Five Stages of demographic transition

Stage 1 High Stationary	Stage 2 Early Expanding	Stage 3 Late Expanding	Stage 4 Low Stationary	Stage 5 Declining
High birth and death rates lead to a low growth rate of the population	A decline in death rate and no change in birth rate leads to a population explosion	The birth rate starts falling with death rates declining rapidly. Population grows at a diminishing rate	Birth rate declines tending to equal the death rate. The stationary growth rate of the population	Death rates exceed birth rates and the population growth declines

Importance of the demographic study:

➤ Demographic data about future population trends are generally required for the formulation of policies with respect to manpower, health, education, etc.

➤ Governments use socioeconomic information to understand the age, racial makeup, and income distribution (among several other variables) in neighbourhoods, cities, states, and nations in order to make better public policy decisions.

➤ Governments keep track of the general fertility rate to determine if their population will grow, shrink, or stay the same size. This determines how healthcare is addressed.

Fertility in India: The total fertility rate is used to measure fertility (TFR). *It is the average number of children a woman will have during her childbearing years* **(TFR) (15-49).**

Interpretation of TFR

If the TFR is 2.1, it means that each generation replaces itself exactly. If the TFR is less than 2.1, the population starts to go down. A stable population is thought to have a total birth rate of 2.1.

India's Total Fertility Rate (TFR) was almost six children per woman in the 1950s, but it is now only 2.2. Based on the TFR level, the Indian government has put states into three groups:

➤ Very high-focus (more than or equal to 3.0), which includes Bihar, Uttar Pradesh, and Meghalaya.

➤ High focus (more than 2.1 and less than 3.0): Madhya Pradesh, Rajasthan, Jharkhand, Chhattisgarh, and Assam.

➤ Non-high focus (less than or equal to 2.1): Panjab

According to the United Nation, India's population will reach 1.66 billion people by 2050 after which it will remain constant and gradually fall. So, spending more on family planning can help to lessen the effects of a fast rise in population. Through Mission Pariwar Vikas, which is being implemented in 13 states, family planning is being integrated into reproductive, maternal, newborn, child, and adolescent health (RMNCH+A).

Family Planning

Family planning is the practice of using safe and effective methods of birth control by couples in order to have the desired number of children in their lifetime and it also helps to maintain the age interval between the children. To enable couples to make an educated, voluntary decision, the National Family Programs aims to provide the right information and assistance on family planning methods.

Family planning Methods: Family planning has undergone a paradigm shift and emerged as a key intervention to reduce maternal and infant mortalities and morbidities. The methods available can be broadly divided into two categories:

➢ Spacing methods

➢ Permanent methods

Spacing Methods: These are the reversible methods of contraception to be used by couples who wish to have children in the future. These include:

Table 2.2 Methods of family planning

Method	Description	How it works?
Oral contraceptives MALA-N" is available free of cost at all public healthcare facilities.	Progestin-only pills are taken orally **once a day** at a fixed time.	The Pill prevents eggs from being released so that the woman cannot become pregnant
Combined Oral Contraceptives (COCs)	It is a combination of Levonorgestrel and ethinyoestradiol with additional ferrous fumarate tablets. The strip also contains additional iron pills to be consumed during the hormonal pill free days (21 hormonal tablets and 7 non-hormonal (iron) tablets)	By preventing or delaying ovulation

Table 2.2 Contd...

Method	Description	How it works?
Emergency Contraceptive Pill EC pills that contain only progestin–Levonorgestrel (1.5mg per tablet)	A progestin-only method. Prevents pregnancy in an emergency situation (unprotected /accidental intercourse) to be taken within 72 hours as a single dose (1.5 mg).	It acts by preventing the implantation of the fertilized ovum into the uterus.
Non Hormonal	Taken twice a week on fixed days for the first three months, followed by once a week thereafter. Centchroman "Chhaya"-once-a-week non-steroidal oral pill has also been recently introduced into the current basket of choices.	It acts by preventing the implantation of the fertilized ovum into the uterus
Hormonal IUD IUCD 380 A, effective up to 10 years, IUCD 375, effective up to 5 years	A small, "T-shaped" copper bearing intra-uterine contraceptive device, popularly known as IUCD, is a small, flexible plastic frame containing coiled copper impregnated with barium sulphate. It is inserted in the uterus by a trained service provider after proper screening and obtaining consent.	It causes changes in the body of the woman that damages the sperm and the egg before they meet.
Injections Available under 'Antara' programme single dose vials (150 mg). Norigynon (Progestrogen and Estrogen). Its effects last for one (1) month. Noristerat (Progestrogen only).Its effects last for two (2) months. Depo Provera (Progestrogen only).Its effects last for three (3) months	**Medroxy Progesterone Acetate (MPA)** Injectable contraceptive MPA is a three-monthly injection containing synthetic hormone progestin and is available at government health facilities under the Antara Programme of National Family Planning Program.	Like the Pill, the substance in the injectable prevents eggs from being released.

Table 2.2 *Contd...*

Method	Description	How it works?
Implants Like the Pill, the substance in the injectable prevents eggs from being released	A thin, flexible plastic rod that releases progestin is inserted under the skin of the upper arm and can prevent pregnancy for up to three years.	Implants work by thickening cervical mucus, making it hard for sperms to pass through.
Vaginal rings	A small ring that contains estrogen and progestin is inserted into the vagina once a month for three weeks of the month.	It releases a continuous dose of the hormone's estrogen and progesterone into the bloodstream to prevent ovaries to release eggs.
Dermal patchs	A thin plastic patch sticks to the skin and releases estrogen and progestin.	It releases estrogen and progestin.
Male Condoms	The Male Condom is a thin rubber sheath that fits over the erect penis. It holds the sperm and prevents it from entering the womb.	It holds the sperm and prevents it from entering the womb and prevent STIs including HIV infection.
Female condoms	The Female Condom is a safe pre-lubricated contraceptive for women. It is made of strong soft rubber	It gently lines the vagina to create a barrier against pregnancy and germs that cause sexually transmitted infections, (e.g. Gonorrhea, Syphilis and HIV/AIDS).

Permanent/Limiting Methods:

- ➢ Male Sterilization (Conventional and Non-Scalpel Vasectomy)
- ➢ Female Sterilization (Minilap and Laproscopic)

Male sterilization (vasectomy)	MALE STERILIZATION VASECTOMY	Vasectomy is a simple operation in which the tubes that carry the sperms in a man are cut and closed. The man still makes semen (the milky liquid) but there are no sperms in it.
Female sterilization (Tubal ligation)	FEMALE STERILIZATION TUBAL LIGATION	Tubal Ligation is an operation in which fallopian tubes that carry the woman's eggs to the womb are cut and blocked.

Family Planning Services: The Government of India provides many family planning services at the village level, state level, and higher levels through ASHAs (Accredited Social Health Activists), health volunteers, nurses, and doctors.

Table 2.3 Types of family planning services provided at different service delivery levels

Service delivery levels			
Delivery points	**Household/ Health post**	**Health centres and rural level**	**Referral hospital**
Type of service	Condoms, oral contraceptives, injections, and single rod implants (Implanon), as well as counselling Mala-D, Mala-N, Ecroz, Khushi, Apsara and Saheli.	Condoms, oral contraceptives, injections, multiple rod implants (Jadelle and Norplants) and Intrauterine contraceptive devices (IUCDs), as well as counselling.	All types of services including Voluntary Surgical Procedures (VSG) and counselling.

Table 2.4 Benefits of family planning

Benefits of Family Planning	
	Protects women's and children's health by reducing high-risk pregnancies and allowing sufficient time between pregnancies. Contraceptive use reduces maternal mortality and improves women's health by preventing unwanted and high-risk pregnancies and reducing the need for unsafe abortions.
	Reduces HIV and AIDS through the prevention of new HIV infections and mother-to-child transmission via increased access to voluntary family planning information, services, and commodities, including condoms.

Table 2.4 *Contd...*

	Decreases abortion Most abortions result from unwanted pregnancies, and significant numbers of maternal deaths can be attributed to unsafe abortions induced by untrained practitioners. Family planning helps mothers prevent such unwanted pregnancies.
	Advances individuals' rights to decide their own family size.
	Improves women's opportunities for education, employment, and full participation in society.
	Reduces poverty by contributing to economic growth at the family, community, and national levels.
	Mitigates the impact of population dynamics on natural resources and state stability.

Role of Pharmacist in family planning: Pharmacists should not miss any opportunity to guide and educate their clients as they are generally the first or only contact of clients with a health professional. The major roles are:

➢ Educating patients regarding safe and effective contraception use, including adverse effects.

➢ Counselling on risks and benefits of different products, and their cost and availability.

➢ Managing logistics and Information Systems (FP-LMIS), which is meant to give ASHAs reliable data on contraceptive demand and distribution.

➢ Providing leaflets containing accurate information about emergency contraception.

➢ Taking part in STD prevention, contraception programs, and providing OTC medication counselling for patients.

➢ Encouraging women to seek medical attention if any unfavourable effects are noticed e.g. change in the bleeding period.

➢ Providing information regarding various FP indemnity schemes.

   • Under section Ia the Government provides indemnity of 2 lakh; if there is death following sterilization (inclusive of death during the process of sterilization operation) in the hospital or within 7 days from the date of discharge from the hospital.

   • Under section Ib, Rs 50 thousand is given; if there is death following sterilization within 8-30 days from the date of discharge from the hospital.

   • Under section Ic, Rs 30 thousand, in case of failure of sterilization.

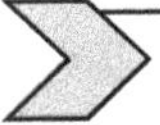 ## 2.2   Maternal and Child Health

Maternal and child health (MCH) care is the health service provided to all women in their reproductive age groups (15 - 49 years), children, school-age population, and adolescents and is listed among the Sustainable Development Goals (SDGs) by the United Nations.

Mother and child as a single unit (Special nature of the group): Mothers and children are regarded as a distinct group and both are considered a single entity for the following reasons:

➢ During the prenatal stage, the foetus is an integral part of the mother. The duration is roughly 280 days. The mother's blood serves as the foetus's sole source of nutrition and oxygen during this stage.

➢ Mother and child health are closely related to one another. Premature birth, stillbirth, and abortion are less likely when a healthy woman gives birth to a healthy child.

➢ Certain diseases, such as syphilis, german measles, etc. are transmitted from the mother to the foetus during pregnancy and are likely to have an impact on the child's health.

➢ The new-born is entirely dependent on the mother for feeding for at least the first six to nine months after birth.

➢ The primary socialization of a child is always initiated by the mother.

➢ The mother also has a strong impact on the child's mental and social development. (Mother deprivation syndrome).

Demographic profile:

➢ In India, women of childbearing age account for 22.8 percent of the population, while children under the age of 15 account for 37.1 percent. Together, they account for 60% of the population.

➢ Mothers and children are the most frequent users of health services, and they also represent a vulnerable or high-risk category. The risk is connected with childbearing in the case of women and growth and development and survival in the case of infants and children.

➢ In the industrialized world, persons over the age of 70 account for half of all deaths, whereas in the developing world, children under the age of five account for the same proportion of deaths.

Major problems: Women and children are responsible for almost half of the disease burden in our country. The major problems are:

➢ Poor reproductive health

➢ Malnutrition

➢ Communicable diseases of childhood: pneumonia, measles, diarrheal diseases, malaria, other vaccine-preventable infections (VPIs), and intestinal parasitic infestations.

These issues contribute to an unacceptable death rate among women in their reproductive years and young children. Safe maternity and early childhood care services are required due to the high Maternal Mortality Rate (MMR) and Infant Mortality Rate (IMR).

The objective of MCH program: The specific objective is

- To reduce maternal, infant, and childhood mortality and morbidity.
- To promote the physical and psychological development of children and adolescents.
- To ensure and promote the health and well-being of mothers and children of all ages by **providing comprehensive, promotive, preventive, curative, and rehabilitative services** so that they attain a high level of health.

Major Domains: The RMNCHA strategy, which was adopted by the Government of India in 2013, takes a 'life-cycle' approach to maternal and child health and is built on the five pillars of *reproductive, maternal, neonatal, child, and adolescent health.*

As a result, India's mother and child health program has moved from a vertical, facility-based, clinical, and doctor-centric model to a decentralized, community-based, participatory, and integrative approach.

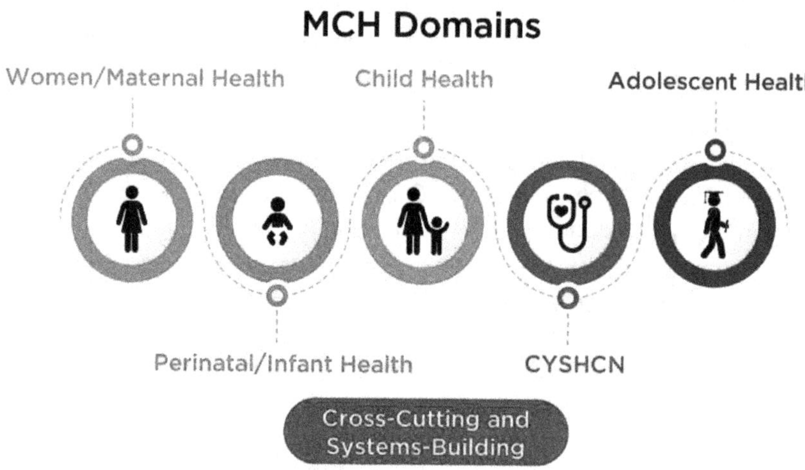

MCH Domains

Figure 2.1 MCH domains

MCH care interventions: Maternal and child health (MCH) programs focus on health issues concerning women, children, and families. The Government of India has demonstrated its commitment and played a proactive leadership role through the national RMNCH+A intervention. The major interventions are shown in the following table:

Table 2.5 Major interventions RMNCH+A

Adolescents & pre-pregnancy	Pregnancy	Mothers	Children	Infants
Family planning **Prevent& manage** sexually transmitted illnesses including HIV Prevention and mother- to-child transmission for HIV and syphilis **Folic acid fortification** and/or supplementation for preventing neural tube defects	**Management of unintended pregnancy** a) Availability and provision of safe abortion care when indicated and legally permitted b) Provision of post abortion care	**Early identification** of maternal Complication **Preventive health check-ups** Counseling on family planning, birth, and emergency preparedness, Birth spacing **Prevention and management of HIV,** including with antireterovirals **Iron and folic acid** to prevent maternal anemia Smoking cessation	**Routine Immunization** and H. influenzae, meningococcal, pneumococcal and Rotavirus vaccines **Treatment** of anaemia **Management** of severe acute malnutrition diarrohea, childhood pneumonia childhood malaria **Vitamin A prophylaxis** from 6 months of age	**Exclusive breastfeeding** within 1 hour of delivery **Breastfeeding**
Cross-cutting community strategies: Home visits for women and children across the continuum of care				

51

Breast Feeding

Breastfeeding is one of the most effective preventive measures a mother takes to protect her health and promote the survival and health of her infant. According to the World Health Organization 'Initiation of breastfeeding should occur within 1 hour of birth, exclusive breastfeeding should be practiced till 6 months of age, and breastfeeding should be continued until 2 years of age at the least.'

WHO actively promotes breastfeeding as the best source of nutrition for infants and children, and is hoping to improve exclusive breastfeeding rates for the first 6 months to at least 50% by 2025.

➢ Exclusive breastfeeding means giving **only breast milk** to an infant. It has the potential to prevent **13% of under-five deaths** globally each year.

➢ Early initiation of breastfeeding within the first hour of birth in addition to exclusive breastfeeding can cut down **22% of all newborn deaths.**

Composition of Breast Milk: Acinar cells or alveolar cells are responsible for the formation of breast milk. In the fourth month of pregnancy, the acinar cells start producing colostrum which is full of nutrients for the new-born. The major constituent is water along with fat, proteins, carbohydrates, vitamins, and minerals. If a baby is only breastfed, no additional fluids are required.

Factors affecting composition: The composition of breast milk varies and changes due to several factors such as:

➢ **Stage of lactation: Colostrum** is a thick yellowish fluid that is produced during the first week after birth, followed by transitional milk during the second week and mature milk thereafter. **Colostrum** production is sufficient to meet the newborn's nutritional and immunological demands. It helps in eliminating neonatal physiological jaundice as it washes away excess bilirubin.

➢ **Breastfeeding session:**

✓ At the beginning of the feed, the baby drinks foremilk that contains more water, less fat, and nutrients, it quenches the thirst of the baby and provides nutrition.

✓ By the end of the breastfeeding session, the milk is called hind milk, which is thicker and has more fat. It helps the baby to gain weight. Both fore milk and hind milk contain lactose that aids in the growth of good bacteria in the digestive system.

The mother shouldn't abruptly stop feeding the baby and let it stop on its own until the infant has consumed the hind milk.

Advantages of Breastfeeding:

For the Infant:

➤ Breast milk is **easily digestible** and free from allergens, unlike cow's milk.

➤ **Protects the child from the gastrointestinal tract:** The presence of *Lactobacillus bifidus* in breast milk prevents colonization of pathogenic bacteria in the gastrointestinal tract, reducing the incidence of diarrhoea. Breast milk has immunoglobulin A, which binds to the invading germs and viruses and prevents the infant's gastrointestinal tract from many infections. **Lactoferrin,** a protein found in breast milk prevents bacteria from multiplying.

➤ **Protects the child from respiratory tract infections: Leukocytes** in breast milk provide protection against common respiratory infections. **Macrophages** produce **interferons** (proteins that are part of your natural defense) that protect the child against common viruses.

➤ **Helps in the growth of newborn:** Breast milk provides the optimum balance of electrolytes and minerals for newborn growth. The levels of nutrients are enough to supply the infant's needs and also spare the infant's kidneys from processing a high renal solute load of unused nutrients. A high level of lactose gives newborns quick access to glucose and promotes rapid brain development. **Linoleic acid** in milk, an essential fatty acid helps in maintaining skin integrity. **Calcium** is regulated better in newborns that are breastfed.

➤ **Prevents excessive weight gain in infants**: Breastfeeding provides the optimal amount of all nutrients and prevents the child from excessive weight gain.

➤ Breastfed children **have better cognitive development** and a higher IQ.

➤ Breastfed babies **have better teeth development** due to jaw movement. Similarly, they **have a lesser risk of dental caries** due to the presence of suitable nutrients in breast milk.

For the Mother:

➤ It lowers the risk of maternal cancers (ovarian and breast cancer)

➤ Oxytocin released during breast feeding helps the uterus to retain back its shape and position.

➤ Breastfeeding empowers women because only women can master it.

➤ It also reduces feeding and preparation time.

➤ It strengthens the bond between the mother and the baby.

➤ Nursing mothers are less likely to become pregnant in the early months (lactational amenorrhea).

➤ It reduces postpartum bleeding and depression.

➤ It helps in faster maternal recovery and post-partum weight loss.

Breast Milk Substitutes: Alternative names: Formula feeding; Bottle feeding; New-born care - infant formula.

Breast milk is a complex nutritional fluid containing antibodies, enzymes, long-chain fatty acids, and hormones, which cannot be added to artificial milk. Breast milk substitutes can be recommended for mothers, who are sick and unable to breastfeed, mothers with twins, or orphaned kids.

Baby formula is a breast milk substitute formulated industrially in accordance with applicable Food and drug standards, to satisfy the normal nutritional requirements of infants up six months of age. It provides a similar number of calories, fat, and protein per ounce as breast milk

Different formulas (Cerelac, Nestum, Farex, Lactogen)

➢ Standard cow's milk-based

➢ Soy-based: Soy-based formulas should be used for infants with galactosemia (a condition in which milk sugar galactose cannot be converted to glucose).

➢ Hypoallergenic formulas (protein hydrolysate formulas)

➢ Lactose-free formulas

Significant issues with the Infant formula:

➢ Poor hygiene in the preparation of infant formula, inadequate cleaning of bottles, and poor storage of infant formula.

➢ Contamination of infant formula with environmental chemicals e.g Fluoridation of milk if constituted with tap water.

➢ Over and under-dilution of infant formula also appears to be common. Under-dilution of infant formula can result in hypernatraemic dehydration and over-dilution in hyponatremia (water intoxication), both of which are potentially fatal.

➢ Increased ear infections, GI disorders, skin conditions, and risk of chronic diseases (diabetes, heart disease, asthma, and some cancers) lower scores on the intelligence test.

➢ **Impact on mothers:** Slower maternal recovery and weight loss, more likely to become pregnant in the early months, post-partum depression, and increased risk of maternal cancers (ovarian and breast cancer).

Bottle feeding disadvantages:

➢ Expensive.

➢ Bottle feeding takes more time for feeding and preparation.

➢ Lower levels of antibodies and nutritional value.

➢ At the risk of swallowing too much air.

- ➢ Increased risk of gas, reflux, and constipation.
- ➢ Proactive mother/baby bonding does not get established.

IMS Act: In 1992, India adopted the Infant Milk Substitutes, Feeding Bottles, and Infant Foods **(IMS)** Act which was strengthened in 2003. The law emphasizes:

- ➢ No promotion to the general public (television advertising, special displays, reductions in pharmacies, etc.).
- ➢ No samples to be given away to the general public.
- ➢ No promotion in health facilities No gifts or samples for health workers.
- ➢ No direct distribution by companies in emergency or crisis situations.
- ➢ No statement of the superiority of breastfeeding on packaging Information provided by companies to health workers.

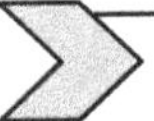

2.3   Overview of Vaccines and Types of Immunity

Immune System: The immune system is designed to defend the body against foreign or dangerous invaders. Such invaders include

- Microorganisms (commonly called germs, such as bacteria, viruses, and fungi
- Parasites (such as worms)
- Cancer cell
- Transplanted organs and tissues

Components of the immune system: The immune system is made up of special organs, cells, and chemicals that fight infection (microbes). The main parts of the immune system are:

- **Adenoids.** Two glands are located at the back of the nasal passage.
- **Bone marrow.** The soft, spongy tissue is found in bone cavities.
- **Peyer patches.** Lymphoid tissue in the small intestine.
- **Spleen.** A fist-sized organ located in the belly (abdominal) cavity.
- **Thymus.** Two lobes join in front of the windpipe (trachea) behind the breastbone.
- **Tonsils.** Two oval masses in the back of the throat.
- **Lymphatic system:** It is a vital part of the immune system along with thymus, bone marrow tonsils, and peyer patches in the small intestine.
- **Lymphatic vessels:** The lymphatic system is a network of lymph nodes connected by lymphatic vessels that helps the body transport microorganisms and dead or damaged cells to be filtered out and destroyed. Acquired immune responses are initiated in the lymph nodes.

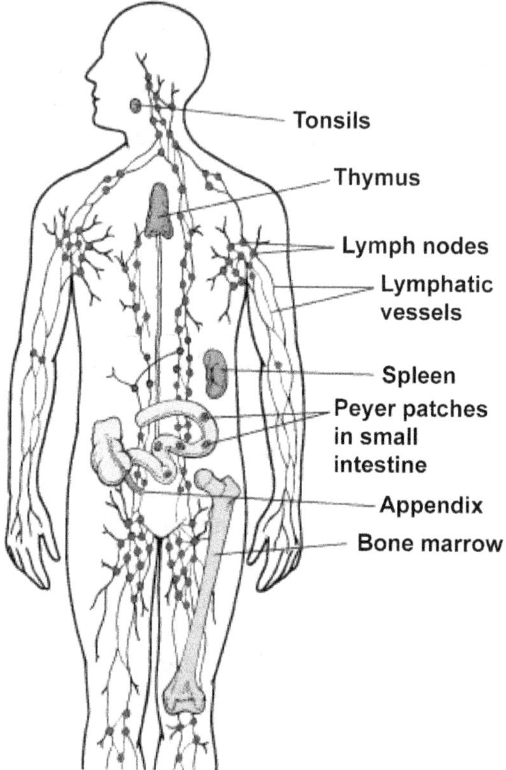

Figure 2.2 Immune system of the body

- **Lymph nodes.** Small organs shaped like beans, are located all over the body and connect via the lymphatic vessels. These are tightly packed with white blood cells.

- Lymph transfers foreign substances (such as bacteria), cancer cells, and dead or damaged cells present in tissues into lymphatic vessels and to lymph nodes for disposal before fluid is returned to the bloodstream. Lymph contains many WBC.

White blood cells: WBC or Leukocytes are important components of the immune system and the body's defense against infections. Blood vessels and lymphatic vessels, which run alongside veins and arteries, transport these cells throughout the body. Whenever they find a target, they multiply and send signals to other cells in the body to do the same. There are several types with different purposes:

Phagocytes are types of white blood cells that are part of our natural immunity, and they work by eating invaders. The four main types of cells which perform phagocytosis are:

- ➤ **Neutrophils**: Neutrophils are the most common and the first responders to an inflammatory response. They digest bad cells and can trap bacteria and stop them from spreading.

- ➤ **Monocytes**: Monocytes are a type of white blood cell that comes from bone marrow. They can become either macrophage cells or dendritic cells when an invading germ or bacteria enters your body. The cells either kill the invader or alert other blood cells to help destroy it and prevent infection.

- ➤ **Macrophages:** They remove dead and dying cells.

- ➤ **Eosinophils:** mainly attach to parasites that are too big to ingest in order to kill them

- ➤ **Mast cells**: Cells in tissues that release histamine and other substances involved in inflammatory and allergic reactions.

- ➤ Dendric cells are derived from white blood cells. They reside in tissues and help T cells recognize foreign antigens

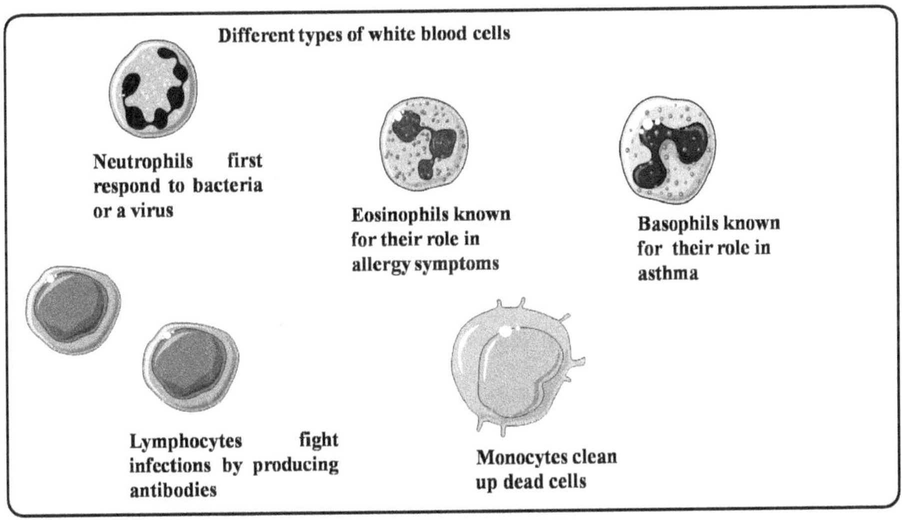

Figure 2.3 Cells involved in imparting immunity

Lymphocytes: Lymphocytes spend most of their lives in the bone marrow and either mature into B cells or migrate to the thymus gland to become T cells. B cells act as the body's military intelligence system, locating targets and directing defenses against them. T cells function similarly to soldiers in that they eliminate intruders discovered by the intelligence system i.e. B cells.

- • **B lymphocytes**: Produce antibodies and help alert the T lymphocytes.

- • **T lymphocytes**: Destroy compromised cells in the body and help alert other leukocytes

Response of the immune system

- When the body senses foreign substances (called antigens), the immune system works to recognize the antigens and get rid of them.

- B lymphocytes are triggered to make antibodies (also called immunoglobulins). These antibodies typically remain in our systems after they are created in case we need to fight the same infection again. This is why a person who contracts an illness, such as chickenpox, will typically not contract it again.

Immunity: The word immunity means the state of protection from infectious diseases through the immune system. Humans have three types of immunity: innate, adaptive, and passive

Innate Immunity: It is the body's first line of defense against invaders including viruses, germs, parasites, and poisons as well as for sensing injuries or trauma e.g. the skin acts as a barrier to block germs from entering the body. Innate immunity is sub-divided into two types:

- ➢ **Non-Specific** innate immunity, is a general resistance offered to all infections.

- ➢ **Specific** innate immunity, where a distinct resistance specific to a microorganism is displayed.

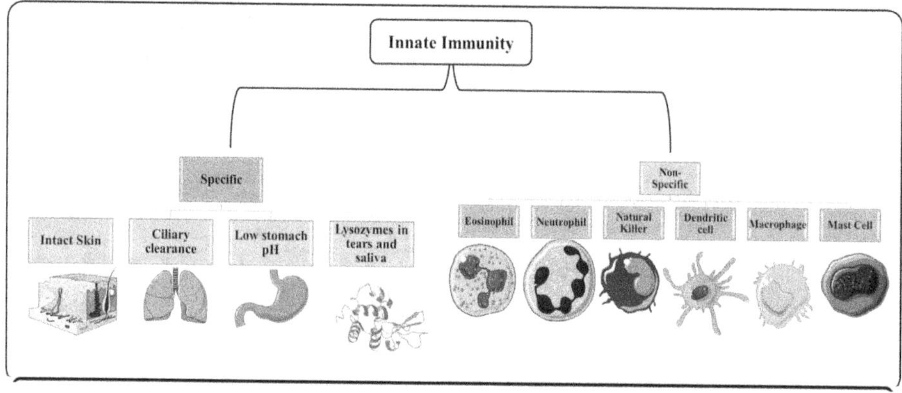

Figure 2.4 Innate immunity

Adaptive Immunity: It gradually develops over the span of a person's life. The body develops adaptive immunity when exposed to a disease or when given a vaccine to prevent it. It can be sub-divided into:

- ➢ **Active immunity: It develops through accidental contact with a disease-causing substance. It can be received through a vaccine and often ensures long-lasting immunity.**

> **Natural:** When there is either a clinical attack of disease e.g. smallpox, chickenpox, rubella, and measles or subclinical infection (e.g. poliomyelitis, diphtheria, cholera, viral hepatitis).

Artificial immunity: This is attained by the administration of vaccines

Passive immunity: It is acquired artificially through deliberate actions. It is briefly present and was "derived" from another source. Passive immunity can occur in a couple of ways:

> **Maternal antibodies:** Unborn and newly born babies are protected by antibodies from the maternal immune system. These antibodies are shared in two ways: across the placenta and in breast milk.

> **Immunoglobulin treatments:** In certain situations, antibodies obtained from animals, from other people, or synthesized in a laboratory can be used to treat individuals at risk of infections.

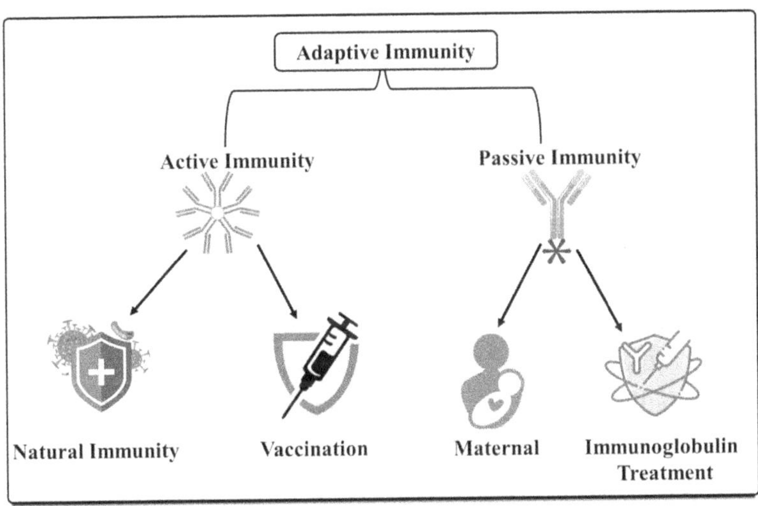

Figure 2.5 Adaptive immunity

Mode of action: Innate immune system activates cells to attack and destroy any invader as the first line of defense followed by informing and modulating the *adaptive* immune response

Vaccines

The term vaccine refers to the **preparation used for immunization i.e. preparation that is used to stimulate the body's immune response and to protect it against diseases.** Once stimulated by a vaccine, the antibody-producing cells, called B cells (B lymphocytes), remain sensitive and ready to respond to the agent if it ever gets entry into the body. So a vaccine provides active immunity to specific harmful agents by stimulating the immune system to attack the agent. A vaccine may also provide passive immunity by developing antibodies.

Vaccines are usually administered by injections (parenteral administration), but some are given orally or even nasally (in the case of flu vaccine).

Vaccination: The act of introducing a vaccine into the body to produce protection from a specific disease. The vaccination uses the body's immune system to increase protection from an infection before coming into contact with that infection

Need for Vaccines: After birth, babies are protected from microorganisms that cause disease for a few weeks. This defense from their mother is passed to the fetus through the placenta. This natural defense quickly loses its effectiveness. So to safeguard the body against diseases, vaccines are administered.

Types of Vaccines:

Four types of vaccines are currently available:

- ➢ **Live virus vaccines** use the weakened (attenuated) form of the virus e.g. measles, mumps, and rubella (MMR) vaccine and varicella (chickenpox) vaccine.

- ➢ **Killed (inactivated) vaccines** are made from a protein or other small pieces taken from a virus or bacteria. Whooping cough (pertussis) vaccine.

- ➢ **Toxoid vaccines** contain a toxin or chemical made by the bacteria or virus e.g. diphtheria and tetanus vaccines.

- ➢ **Biosynthetic vaccines** contain manmade substances that are very similar to pieces of the virus or bacteria e.g. Hepatitis B.

Immunological Mechanism of vaccination

- • Vaccines "teach" the body how to defend itself when germs, such as viruses or bacteria, invade it.

- • Vaccines expose the body to a very small, very safe number of viruses or bacteria that have been weakened or killed.

- • The immune system then learns to recognize and attack the infection if the person is exposed to it later in life.

- • As a result, the person will not become ill or may have a milder infection. This is a natural way to deal with infectious diseases.

Immunization: Around 2.5 million deaths are avoided annually due to vaccination initiatives. According to the National immunization programme, a series of immunizations are administered from infancy until adulthood. Major immunization programmes are:

Table 2.6 Immunisation at various ages of life

Age	Disease to protect against	
Pregnancy	Tetanus + diptheria + whooping cough (pertussis) Influenza	
6-9 weeks weeks	Rotavirus (first dose must be given before 15 weeks) Around 2.5 million deaths are avoided annually due to vaccination initiatives. According to the National immunization programme, a series of immunizations are administered. From infancy until adulthood, people receive various immunizations from infancy until adulthood. Diphtheria + tetanus + whooping cough (pertussis) + polio + hepatitis B + *Haemophilusinfluenzae* type b (Hib) Pneumococcal disease	
3 months	Rotavirus (second dose must be given before 25 weeks) Diphtheria + tetanus + whooping cough (pertussis) + polio + hepatitis B + *Haemophilusinfluenzae* type b (Hib)	
5 months	Diphtheria + tetanus + whooping cough (pertussis) + polio + hepatitis B + *Haemophilus influenzae* type b (Hib) Pneumococcal disease	
12 months	Measles + mumps + rubella +Pneumoccal	
15 months	Haemophilusinfluenzae type B (Hib) Measles + mumps + rubella Chickenpox (varicella)	

Table 2.6 *Contd...*

Age	Disease to protect against	
4 years	Diphtheria + tetanus + whooping cough + polio	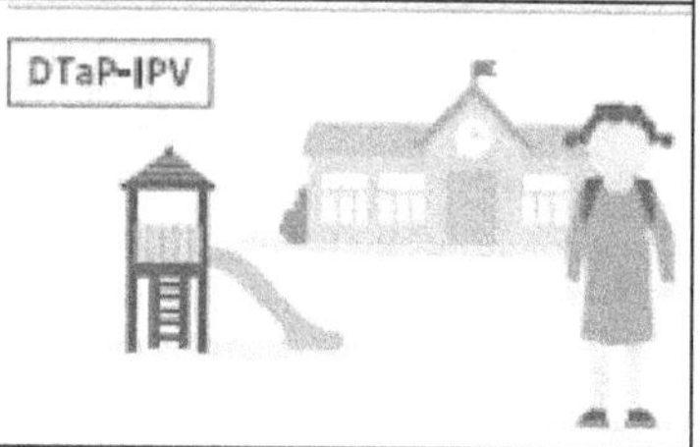 DTaP-IPV
11 + 12 years	Tetanus + diphtheria + whooping cough Human papillomavirus (HPV)	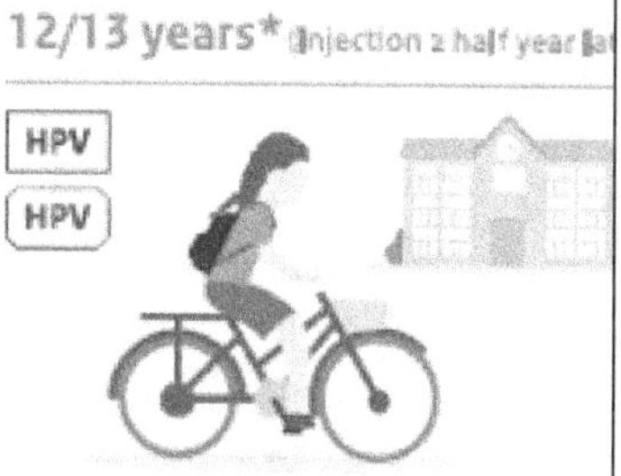 12/13 years* Injection a half year la HPV HPV

Table 2.7 Flagship Immunization Programs in India

1978	Expanded Programme of Immunization	Launch of the Immunization Programme in India
1985	Universal Immunization Programme UIP	prevents mortality and morbidity in children and pregnant women **against 12 vaccine-preventable diseases** Diphtheria, Whooping cough, tetanus, polio, tuberculosis, hepatitis B, meningitis and pneumonia, Haemophilus influenza type B infections, Japanese encephalitis (JE), rotavirus vaccine, pneumococcal conjugate vaccine (PCV) and measles-rubella (MR).
2015	Mission Indradhanush	Special drives in four districts
2017	Intensified Mission Indradhanush (IMI)	Greater focus was given to urban areas which were one of the gaps of Mission Indradhanush.
2019-20	Indradhanush Intensified Mission 2.0	Full immunization coverage in 272 districts spread over 27 States.
2021	Indradhanush Mission Intensified 3.0	IMI 3.0 was the children and pregnant women who had missed their vaccine doses during the Covid-19 pandemic.
2021-22	Indradhanush Mission Intensified 4.0	Routine Immunization (RI) services reach unvaccinated and partially vaccinated children and pregnant women.

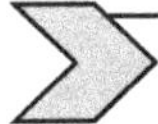 ## 2.4   Effect of Environment on Health

Water Pollution

Water pollution is the contamination of water sources by substances that make the water unusable for drinking, domestic use, food production, recreational purposes, and other activities. **The main water pollutants include bacteria, viruses, parasites, fertilizers, pesticides, pharmaceutical products, nitrates, phosphates, fecal waste, and even radioactive substances.**

All forms of pollution eventually make their way to water pollution e.g. Air pollution settles onto lakes and oceans. Land pollution can seep into an underground stream, then into a river, and finally into the ocean.

Water pollution is one of the leading causes of many diseases like cholera, diarrhea, malaria, and dengue. The burden of water-related diseases falls disproportionately on developing countries and particularly on children under five, with 30% of deaths of these children due to inadequate access to safe drinking water and sanitation.

Safe drinking water

> Water is considered the main developmental pillar under SDG6 by the UN which states '**water sustains life but clean drinking water defines Civilization'**

> Water is a basic human right and access to clean, safe drinking water (potable water) is a fundamental indicator of a society's health and well-being

> **Safe drinking water is the water that is safe for drinking, food preparation personal hygiene, and washing and must meet chemical, biological, and physical quality standards.**

> Access to clean drinking water reduces health risks and frees-up time for education and other productive activities, as well as increases the productivity of the labor force. improving the quality of surface waters benefits the environment (e.g. functioning of ecosystems; biodiversity), So safe water has the potential to decrease the burden of disease and improve public health which results in economic, social, financial, and environmental benefits

Waterborne Diseases

Waterborne diseases are caused by microscopic organisms, like viruses and bacteria that are ingested through contaminated water or by coming into contact with feces. In all water-borne diseases, diarrhea is the common symptom and biggest cause of death among children under five. Diarrhea kills more children than malaria, AIDS, and measles together.

Following are the seven waterborne diseases that affect the community due to the consumption of contaminated water:

1. **Amoebiasis:** It is an intestinal disease caused by a tiny parasite called *Entamoeba histolytica* that spread through human feces. Often there are no symptoms, but sometimes it causes diarrhea and weight loss.

2. **Cholera:** The disease is spread through water contaminated with bacteria; *Vibrio cholera* and causes severe dehydration and diarrhea. Cholera can be fatal within days or even hours of exposure to the bacteria, but only 1 in 10 people develop life-threatening symptoms.

3. **Dysentery:** An intestinal infection caused by *E. histolytica and Shigella.* It is characterized by severe diarrhea as well as blood or mucus in the stool. Diarrhea may lead to dehydration, so quick fluid replacement is required to overrule the risk to life.

4. **Giardiasis:** *Giardia* is a tiny parasite (germ) that causes the diarrheal disease giardiasis. This waterborne disease spreads through contaminated water of ponds and streams, but it can also be found in a town's water supply, swimming pools, etc. The infection clears up after a few weeks but people experience intestinal problems for years

5. **Hepatitis A:** Hepatitis A is a liver infection caused by the Hepatitis A virus. The virus is transmitted through the ingestion of contaminated food and water or through direct contact with an infectious person.

6. **Salmonellosis/Typhoid Fever:** Typhoid fever is rare in industrialized countries; it is common in very poor parts of developing countries. It is thought that up to 20 million people around the world get sick every year. It is very contagious and spreads through contaminated food, unsafe water, and poor sanitation. Undercooked meat, egg products, fruits, and vegetables can carry the disease. Most people don't develop complications, but children, pregnant women, older adults, and people with weakened immune systems are most at risk.

7. **Escherichia coli (E. coli) infections:** The bacteria are found in and around unsafe water sources where humans and cattle coexist. Symptoms of dangerous strains of *E. coli* are similar to that of dysentery and other waterborne diseases.

Source of Water pollution

1. **Point source pollution:** The discharge of pollutants is from a single identifiable source e.g. municipal sources, industrial sources, etc.

2. **Non-point source pollution:** The discharge of pollutants from random or scattered sources e.g. construction sites, agricultural sites, acid rain, animal waste, etc.

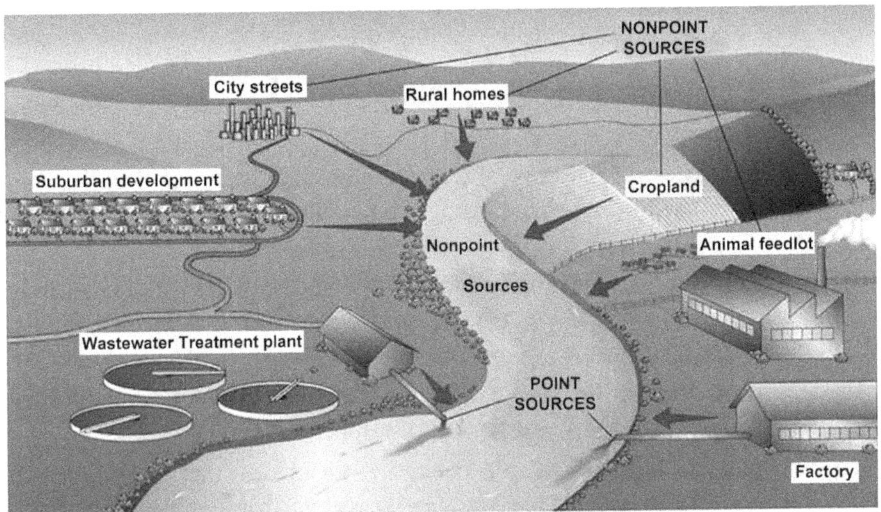

Figure 2.6 Sources of water pollution

Causes of Water pollution:

The main water pollutants include bacteria, viruses, parasites, fertilizers, pesticides, pharmaceutical products, chemicals, plastic, fecal waste, and even radioactive substances. These pollutants are often invisible pollutants as they usually do not change the color of the water. Depending upon the pollutants, different types of contamination are:

(a) **Microbial contamination:** It is responsible for 80% of sickness in underdeveloped countries and caused due to the accidental introduction of disease-causing micro-organisms including bacteria, viruses, and protozoa from raw sewage and animal waste.

(b) **Organic matter (Oxygen-depleting waste):** Organic matter present in water is degraded by aerobic microorganisms. The microorganisms need oxygen to break down the organic waste and it is known as BOD (biochemical oxygen demand). If a large amount of waste is present, then BOD is more which leads to depletion of oxygen in the water.

(c) **Water-soluble inorganic chemicals:** The elements like lead, mercury, cadmium, and arsenic adversely affect humans and animals e.g. cadmium causes Itai-Itai disease, and mercury causes Minamata disease.

(d) **Suspended solids:** The presence of suspended solids in water bodies causes the water to become turbid, which prevents the aquatic plants and animals from receiving enough sunlight, disrupting the balance of the aquatic ecosystem

(e) **Industrial waste:** Industries are major contributors to water pollution. Some industries do not have proper waste management systems and their toxic industrial waste is dumped into nearby freshwater systems which makes water unsafe for human consumption, and also increases the temperature of freshwater systems making it dangerous for many water organisms.

(f) Marine dumping: Many countries throughout the world collect and dump household garbage into oceans which contributes to water pollution.

(g) Sewage and wastewater: Even after treatment, harmful chemicals, germs, and pathogens can be present in sewage and wastewater and pollute water.

(h) Oil leaks and spills: Large oil spills and leaks, though, unintentional, are a significant source of water pollution.

(i) Pesticides: Agricultural practices use pesticides that seep into the groundwater, rivers streams, and finally oceans, causing water pollution.

(j) Global warming: Air pollution and deforestation cause global warming that indirectly contributes to pollution, The rise in water temperatures reduces oxygen content and may kill water-dwelling animals. When large die-offs occur, it further pollutes the water supply and worsens the problem.

Effects of water pollution: Pollution of water affects both humans and aquatic life. Most water sources close to cities and urban centers are polluted by garbage and the dumping of chemicals, legally or illegally. Deteriorating water quality is damaging the environment, health conditions, and the global economy. Below are some of the adverse effects of polluting water bodies.

The Impact on Human Health:
- Lack of potable water leads to increased infant mortality as the diarrheal diseases linked to lack of hygiene caused the death of about 1000 children a day worldwide.
- Drinking or consuming polluted water can cause stomach problems, poisoning, and death, as well as long-term toxicity and neurological problems from more significant chemical pollution.
- Human diseases are most commonly caused by waterborne pathogens. Giardia, typhoid, and cholera are among the diseases spread by contaminated water.
- Chemical pollutants in water on coming into contact with our skin while swimming or doing household work can cause various skin diseases.

The Impact on the environment:
- Pollution disrupts the food chain by moving toxins from one level in the chain to higher levels.

➢ Nutrient pollution destroys the ecosystem, for example, Agricultural sewage dumping by introducing nutrients such as nitrates and phosphates leads to an excessive increase in algae, which depletes the water of oxygen, thereby leading to the death of fish and other aquatic life.

➢ Marine life is also threatened by debris and litter. Plastics take up to 500 years to degrade and have even formed "plastic islands" in oceans.

➢ Pollution harms aquatic life. In contaminated water, animals and plants may die or not reproduce.

The Impact on the Economy:

➢ According to the World Bank report, heavily polluted water is reducing economic growth in some countries. Health expenses related to water-borne diseases are estimated at 470-610 billion rupees per year.

➢ When an aquatic ecosystem is damaged, commercial fishing and aquaculture are likely to be less profitable. Water pollution also results in damage to recreational facilities, particularly around freshwater lakes and major beaches, and reduces revenue.

➢ Water purification costs, including treatment and inspection, are a burden on municipal budgets.

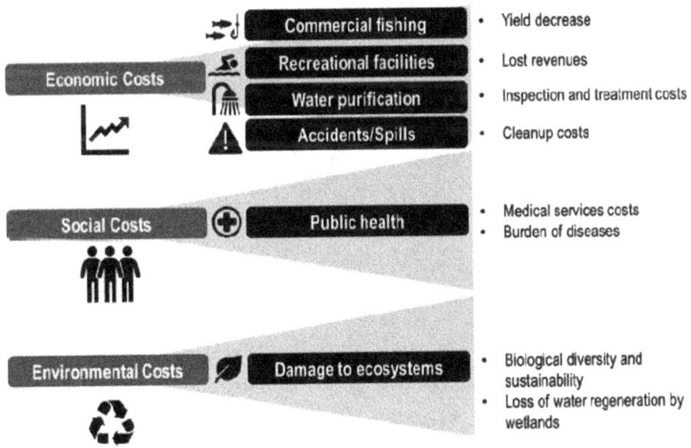

Figure 2.7 Impact of water pollution on society and environment

Prevention and control of water pollution

➢ Encouraging people to plant more trees near bodies of water so that the trees can stop the erosion that washes pollution into the water.

➢ Growing 'Water Hyacinth' that absorbs dissolved toxic substances like cadmium and mercury from water bodies may help in removing pollutants from water.

- The waste should be disposed of carefully, it should not be dumped directly into water bodies, without proper waste treatment.
- Sewage treatment plants and wastewater treatment plants in industries should be established to treat the water.
- Using natural fertilizers and pesticides as substitutes for chemical ones is good for plants and water.
- Chemical processes such as coagulation, ion exchange method, reverse osmosis, etc. will greatly reduce the level of water pollution.
- Public awareness programs for the conservation of resources may help to reduce the consumption of water in our daily activities and reuse water whenever possible to reduce the overall level of pollution.
- Household chemicals, cleaning agents, and unused/ expired medicines should not be disposed into the kitchen sinks or toilets.
- Buy products that are safe and environmentally friendly. Emphasis should be on using detergents and dish cleaners that are free from phosphates.
- Make Swachh Bharat Abhiyan a success by making India completely open and defecation-free.
- Dumping of waste in rivers and other water sources should be prohibited.

Air Pollution

- Air is called polluted if there is an undesirable visible or invisible change in its normal composition due to the presence of gases, dust, fumes, smoke, chemical particulates, or odor in excessive concentrations that can have harmful effects on humans, animals, plants, land, buildings, and water resources.
- Air pollution caused 1.67 million deaths in India in 2019. Fine particulate matter (PM2.5) continues to cause the most substantial health impacts.
- According to the World Health Organization, Delhi had the worst air of 1,600 cities worldwide. Thirteen Indian cities had PM 2.5 levels higher than the WHO recommended guideline of 25, with Delhi's level at 153.

PM 2.5: PM is the abbreviation for particulate matter. Particulate matter 2.5 is a term used to describe microscopic particles or droplets in the air that are less than 2.5 microns in size. PM 2.5 in the air decrease visibility and make the air appear hazy. A high concentration of fine particulate matter (PM2.5) in the air can be harmful to people's health.

Types of Air Pollutants: There are two types of pollutants in the air:

1. Primary Air Pollutants
2. Secondary Air Pollutants

Table 2.8 Types of air pollution

Primary pollutants	Secondary pollutants
Pollutants that are emitted directly from human or natural activities, The source of origin can be identified	Secondary pollutants are formed when primary pollutants react with atmospheric moisture.
Primary pollutants are carbon monoxide, sulfur oxides, nitrogen oxides, fluorides, chlorofluorocarbons, particulate matter, hydrocarbons, and other pollutants are examples.	Secondary pollutants are carbonic acid, nitric acid, sulphuric acid, etc. Classical smog (London smog), peroxy acyl nitrate (PAN), Photochemical smog (Los Angeles smog), acid rain

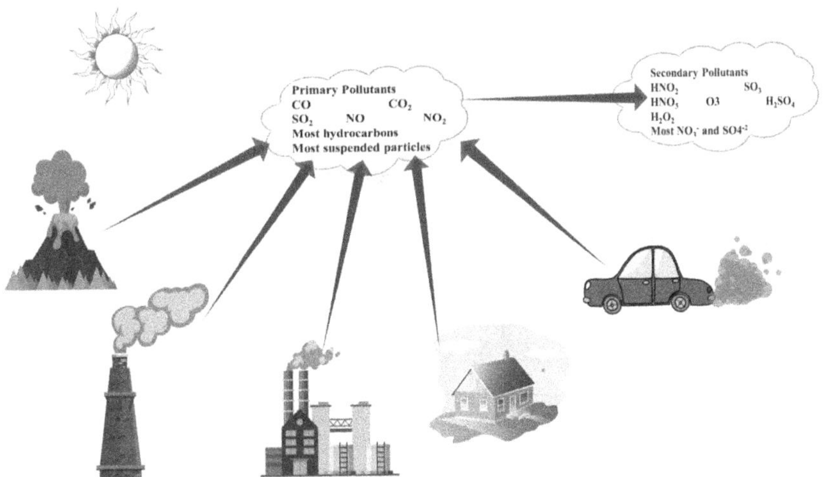

Figure 2.8 Sources and types of Air Pollution

Causes of Air Pollution: Air pollution is a toxic mix of natural and man-made pollutants. It is caused by a variety of factors, including natural sources like forest fires and volcano eruptions. However, man-made factors are the major cause of air pollution worldwide. Vehicle emissions, fuel oils, natural gas used to heat homes, by-products of manufacturing and electricity generation, particularly coal-fueled power plants, and fumes from the chemical industry are the main sources of human-made air pollution.

Sources of the outdoor air pollution

- **Dust**: Dust storms, wind, volcanoes, cars, mining, and other things increase dust in the air

- **Automobiles**: When petrol and diesel are burned in cars, harmful gases are emitted into the air. Automobiles are a major source of greenhouse gases like hydrocarbons, CO, CO_2, and sulfur oxides and cause serious health problems

- **Industries:** Industries such as pharmaceuticals, fertilizers, insecticides, and chemicals emit harmful gases into the atmosphere.

- ➢ **Agriculture:** Plants, pollen grains, pesticides, and gases emitted by decomposing organic matter in soils, such as methane, and ammonia pollute the air.

- ➢ **Ionizing radiations**: Ionizing radiations include alpha particles, beta particles, and gamma rays. They are discharged into the atmosphere during the testing of nuclear weapons and explosions.

- ➢ **Freons** and other chlorine-fluorine carbons used as refrigerants, coolants, and filling agents in aerosol products pollute the environment.

- ➢ **Smoke:** Burning of agricultural waste, solid wastes, and other wastes generates smoke and pollutes the environment.

Sources of the indoor Air pollution

- ➢ **Tobacco smoke:** It is either smoke from burning cigarettes or smoke exhaled by smokers.

- ➢ **Biological Pollutants:** These include allergens such as pollen from plants, hair from pets, fungi, and some bacteria.

- ➢ **Radon**: It is a gas that is naturally emitted from the ground. Radon can be trapped in the basements of buildings and homes. The gas is known to cause cancer after exposure over a period.

- ➢ **Carbon Monoxide:** It is a poisonous gas with no color or smell. Carbon monoxide is produced when fuels such as gas, oil, coal, or wood do not fully burn.

- ➢ **Domestic Sources:** Painting walls, burning cow dung and garbage adds to an unpleasant odor in the air, creating health problems.

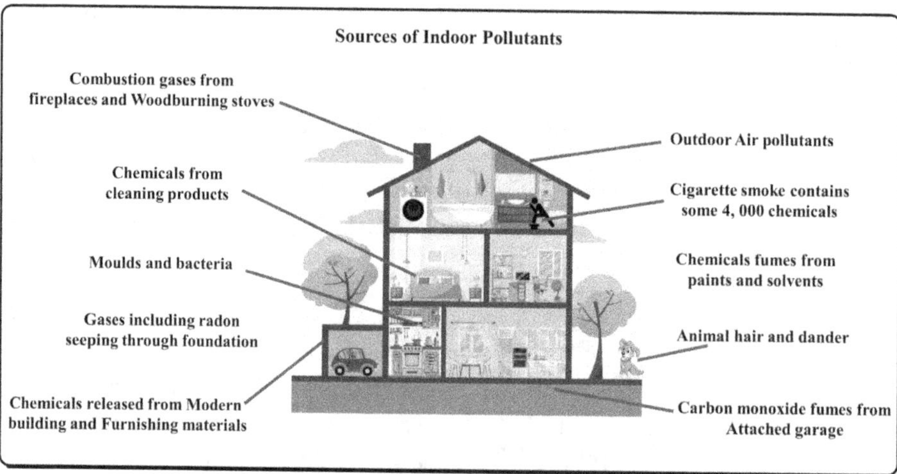

Figure 2.9 Sources of indoor Air pollution

Specific phenomenon related to air pollution:

- ➢ **Smog effect**: When a dense dark fog settles over cities and fields, the smog effect occurs. Smog is produced by industrial and urban activity. It contains a variety of contaminants such as pollens, dust, nitrogen dioxide, ammonia, sulphur dioxide, and other toxic volatile chemicals.

- ➢ **Depletion of the ozone Layer:** Ozone layer depletion is the thinning of the ozone layer present in the upper atmosphere. The ozone layer helps in shielding the harmful ultraviolet rays of the sun. It has the potential to absorb around 97-98% of the harmful ultraviolet radiations coming from the sun that can damage life on earth.

- ➢ Air pollution is responsible for the ozone hole. The chemical substances which are responsible for the depletion of the earth's protective ozone layer are called ozone-depleting substances (ODS). The principal source of ozone depletion is refrigerants such as hydro chlorofluorocarbons, and chlorofluorocarbons. This depletion allows the sun's harmful UV rays to penetrate the atmosphere, causing skin problems and visual problems among the general public.

- ➢ **Acid rain**: Combustion of fossil fuels generates nitrogen oxide and sulfur dioxide, causing acid rain. When water droplets touch pollutants, they become acidic and fall into acid rain, which harms the environment and surfaces.

- ➢ **The Greenhouse Effect:** It is the process through which thermal radiation from a planet's surface is absorbed by greenhouse gases (CO_2, methane, nitrous oxide, and water vapors) in the atmosphere and re-radiated in all directions. The molecules of these gases emit heat energy. This cycle is repeated several times, resulting in the greenhouse effect. Increased amounts of greenhouse gases have resulted in significantly warming of the environment. Deforestation causes CO_2 levels to rise because fewer trees are present to absorb CO_2. Additionally, human activities contribute to the increase in atmospheric CO_2, which increases the greenhouse effect and, as a result, causes global warming.

- ➢ **Global warming:** The gradual increase in the average temperature of the earth's atmosphere is called global warming. Global warming can cause sea levels to rise and affect rainfall patterns, agriculture, forests, plants, and animals.

Indicators of Air Pollution: The indicators of air pollution are sulphur dioxide, carbon monoxide, oxides of nitrogen, lead, and suspended particles (expressed as mg or µg/cubic meter of air). *The smoke index or soiling index* is also used as an indicator of air pollution. In it air is filtered through the paper tape and the density is measured by a photoelectric meter. The smoke index of air quality shows daily, weekly and seasonal variation. To measure the air quality two international centers in London and Washington, three regional centers in Nagpur, Tokyo, and Moscow respectively, and laboratories in big cities have been established. These issue warnings whenever needed. In India, the National Environmental Engineering Research Institute (NEERI) at Nagpur is a WHO regional centre for air quality monitoring. Other big cities also have laboratories for the same.

Bad smells made by factories, garbage, or sewer systems are also considered air pollution. These odors are less serious but still unpleasant.

Effect of air pollution on health and environment:

Health effects: Air pollution leads to a wide range of health effects. Nearly 2.5 million people die worldwide each year from the effects of outdoor or indoor air pollution.

1. **Short-term effects**, which are temporary, include illnesses such as pneumonia or bronchitis, and discomforts such as irritation to the nose, throat, eyes, or skin. It can also cause headaches, dizziness, and nausea.

2. **Long-term effects** of air pollution can last for years or for an entire lifetime. They can even lead to a person's death. Long-term health effects from air pollution include heart disease, lung cancer, and respiratory diseases such as emphysema (shortness of breath), and birth defects. Air pollution can also cause long-term damage to people's nerves, brain, kidneys, liver, and other organs.

3. **Depletion of the ozone layer** exposes humans to harmful ultraviolet rays which cause skin diseases, cataracts, cancer, impaired immune system, etc

4. **Acid rain** does not affect directly but sulfur dioxide particles can cause asthma and bronchitis, and nitrogen oxides increase ground-level ozone formation which causes chronic pneumonia.

5. **Global warming** can cause the spread of infectious diseases such as dengue fever, malaria, and cholera, as well as an increase in the risk of cardiovascular disease.

Effect on the environment:

1. **On Plants:** Sulphur dioxide, hydrogen halides, hydrogen fluoride, and Smog gases, etc may cause leaf injury. The Earth's surface is harmed by acid rain, climate change, and smog. Contaminated water and gases penetrate into the ground, altering soil composition. This has a direct impact on the composition of the harvested crops as it alters the crop cycles.

2. **Effect on works of art:** Air pollution also has a **deleterious effect on works of art.** In India, the discoloration of the Taj Mahal at Agra is an example of the influence of air pollution.

Control and prevention of Air Pollution: Following measures may prevent air pollution:

➢ Reusing and recycling products.

➢ Usage of public transport and carpooling.

➢ Switching off the lights when they're not in use, electricity is produced from the combustion of fossil fuels, which leads to air pollution. Therefore, saving electricity is an effective way of preventing air pollution. The use of energy-efficient gadgets such as CFLs also helps to reduce pollution.

➢ Avoiding the burning of garbage and smoking: Avoiding these activities and spreading awareness of their negative consequences can help in the prevention of air pollution.

➢ Avoiding the use of firecrackers can help prevent air pollution.

➢ PUC certifications for automobiles.

➢ Planting trees in places with high pollution levels.

➢ Industries should upgrade and maintain existing equipment to reduce pollutant emissions.

➢ Utilization of clean energy resources like solar and wind energy.

➢ Use of ultraviolet radiation in operation theatre reduces the bacterial count. Wet cleaning of floors is better than sweeping. The application of oil to floors of hospital wards reduces the bacterial count.

➢ Using dust control equipment like mechanical dust collectors, and scrubbers.

Legislation:

➢ In India, the **'Smoke Nuisance Act'** is effective in big cities. The vehicles must be checked at regular intervals (6 months) for proper maintenance so that they cause minimum pollution (PUC certificate).

➢ The government of India launched a flagship program named **National Clean Air Program (NCAP)** in 2019, to prepare clean air action plans with an objective to reduce PM 2.5 pollution by 20-30% by 2024 as compared to 2017, in 122 cities.

Noise Pollution

➢ Noise pollution, also known as environmental noise or sound pollution, is the loud displeasing, and undesirable sound. It is one of the major environmental issues in India but sadly many are unaware of the hazards it can cause. According to World Health Organization ", noise must be recognized as a major threat to human health.

➢ The standard unit 1 decibel (dB) is the amount of sound that the average person can hear. A normal, healthy individual may tolerate 80 to 90 dB without suffering ear damage. Noise pollution is a result of sound levels above 80 decibels.

Table 2.9 Classification of sound in decibels

Sound	Decibel level
Normal Talking	40 Db
Trains	75 Db
Whisper	20 Db
Air conditioners	60 dB
Aircraft	120 Db
Heavy vehicles	90 Db
Atomic Explosion	200 Db
If sound is at 80 db or more it causes pollution.	

Causes of Noise Pollution

➢ Noise pollution is more common in the workplace than in the general environment. It can be spread by sounds generated by human activities such as loudspeakers, road processions, festive-time expressions of enjoyment by fireworks, and high volume of the music system.

➢ **Outdoor noise pollution:** Transport systems and heavy traffic (heavy vehicles, railroads, locomotive engines, automobiles, loud horns, sound generation while speeding and braking, aircraft, industries (noise of machines), mines (explosions, cutters) Construction of buildings, overpasses, roadways etc.

➢ **Domestic:** The average level of background noise in a normal home nowadays ranges between 40 and 50 decibels. The household power generators and home appliances such as electric chimneys, mixer grinders, air conditioners, and high-volume television and music system may contribute to noise pollution.

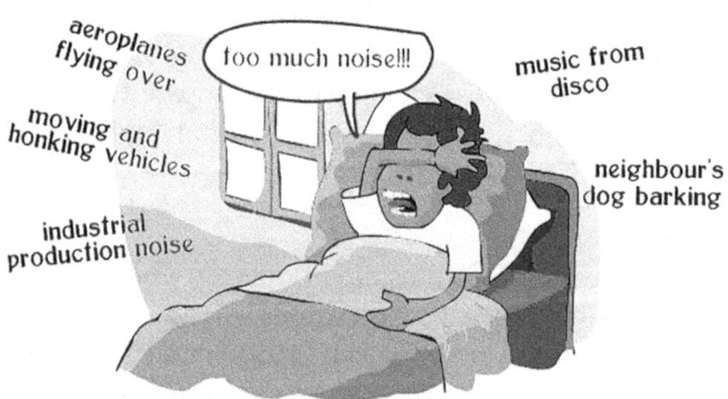

Figure 2.10 Types of noise pollution

Health effects caused by noise pollution: Noise pollution is associated with several health conditions, including:

➢ Interferes with normal activities, such as sleep or conversation, and produces restlessness, anxiety, irritation, tiredness, fatigue, and stress, so affecting an individual's quality of life.

➢ Behavioral annoyance, anxiety, irritation, tiredness, and stress due noise induced sleeplessness.

➢ Repeated exposures to high noise levels can contribute to **cardiovascular disorders in humans that include** hypertension, high-stress levels, and increased **incidence of coronary artery disease**.

➢ **Auditory disturbances like** tinnitus, buzzing in the ears, and temporary/permanent hearing loss depend upon exposure to noise.

➢ Reduces learning and reading skills, decreases work efficiency, and may lead to temporary or permanent deafness due to continuous exposure of ears to mobiles and vehicles.

➢ Noise pollution is also associated with **severe depression, and panic attacks.**

Prevention and Control of Noise Pollution:

1. **Education and Awareness**: Education on noise pollution as a health and community risk is the best control measure. Noise pollution awareness programs should be carried out.

2. **Prevention:**

   ✓ The manufacturers may be encouraged to design quieter appliances, equipment, tools, and machines. The buyer should also check and enquire about the sound of various appliances and machines. Regular servicing and lubrication of the machinery should be done to minimize noise generation.

   ✓ Roadway noise can be efficiently reduced by designing better roads and vehicle tyres, using noise barriers, regulating vehicle speeds, using traffic controls that smooth vehicle flow to decrease braking and acceleration, and routinely servicing cars.

3. **Legislation**: Regulatory measures like restriction on the use of loudspeakers in residential areas, hospitals, and near schools and public places. Factories and industries should be located far from the residential areas. Further, legislation should be enacted to seek compensation for noise-induced hearing loss.

4. **Reduction:** Noise pollution can be reduced by using heavy curtains on the windows and doors, soundproof walls and tiles to absorb sounds, and by wearing ear plugs in noisy places for protection, playing and listening to radio, TV, and music systems on low volume. Planting bushes and trees in and around sound-generating sources.

Occupational Diseases

> Occupational diseases are bad health conditions in humans whose occurrence or severity is connected to factors on the job or in the work environment. The severity of any such diseases depends on the job environment, exposure intensity, and worker sensitivities. Every year, about two million individuals are killed at work.

> The occupational disease can cause death/permanent disability if not prevented or left untreated.

> It was found that 745,000 deaths from ischemic heart disease and stroke events in 2016 were due to exposure to long working hours.

> Occupational hazards that are of a traumatic nature (such as falls from rooftops) are not considered occupational diseases.

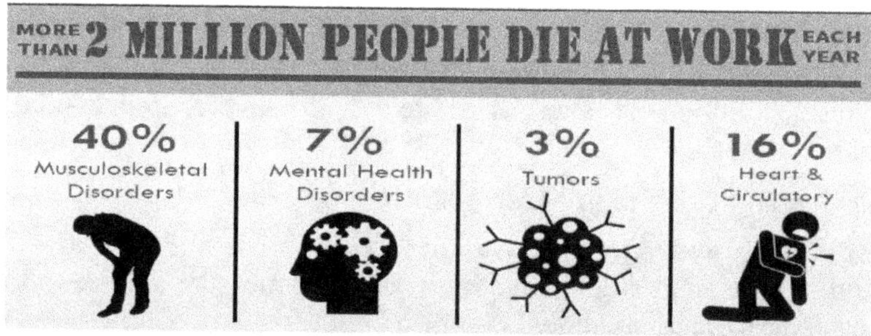

Figure 2.11 Disease burden of occupational illnesses

Factors affecting Occupational Diseases: Following are the various factors that contribute to occupational diseases:

Table 2.10 Factors affecting occupational diseases

Physical	Heat, cold, light Noise, Radiation heat hyperpyrexia, exhaustion, fainting, cramps, burns, trench Foot, frostbite, work-related cataracts, hearing loss, cancers, aplastic anemia
Chemical	Solvents, pesticides, heavy metals, dust

Table 2.10 *Contd...*

Biological	**Bacteria, viruses, mycobacterium** Tuberculosis, hepatitis B Virus, HIV, covid19
Ergonomic **And Mechanical**	**Improperly designed tools or work areas** These mainly cause work accidents and injuries rather than occupational diseases.
Psychosocial **Stressors**	**Overwork, inadequate personal support** Ischemic heart disease and stroke

Common occupational diseases in India: Asthma, COPD, dermatitis, and musculoskeletal disorders are considered common occupational disorders. The 3rd schedule of the **Indian Factories Act**-1948 provides a list of occupational diseases. A few of those include:

> **Poisoning by metals** and compounds such as lead, tetra-ethyl lead, phosphorous, mercury, manganese, arsenic, nitrous fumes, carbon bisulphide, benzene, their nitro or amino derivatives: The workers of industries related with storage batteries, glass, shipbuilding, printing, and potteries, rubber may suffer with lead poisoning.

> **Silicosis:** Silicosis is caused by crystalline silica (SiO_2) in workers engaged in mining (coal, mica, gold, silver, lead, zn), stone cutting and shaping, sandblasting (building and construction), glass and ceramics manufacture, iron and steel industry. It takes 7–10 years to develop silicosis after prolonged exposure to higher concentrations of dust. It is a progressive disease and converts to TB.

> **Skin Cancer and dermatitis due to mineral oils:** Long-term outdoor laborers including those exposed to harsh chemicals, develop skin diseases. Hairdressers, caterers, healthcare workers, printers, metalworkers, and motor mechanics often get occupational skin diseases. The causative factors are chemicals and wet hands at work and major symptoms are urticaria, skin cancer, and eczema.

➤ **Asbestosis:** It is a chronic lung disease that develops on long exposure to the inhalation of asbestos fibers. It is common among workers involved in the mining of asbestos from natural deposits, processing of asbestos minerals, manufacturing of asbestos products, construction industry, mechanics, insulation workers, sheet metal workers, plumbers, pipe fitters, cement workers, etc.

It is characterized by scar-like tissue formed in the lungs (pulmonary fibrosis). The symptoms develop over a long period of time. People with fully developed asbestosis have shortness of breath, cough, chest pain, reduced lung function, finger clubbing, and bluish skin coloration.

➤ **Coal miners' pneumoconiosis:** Pneumoconiosis is a lung disease that results from the inhalation of various types of inorganic dust, such as silica, asbestos, coal, talc, and china clay.

➤ **Occupational COVID-19 exposure:** After the COVID-19 pandemic of 2020 coronavirus has been added to the list of potential occupational diseases. Doctors and other healthcare workers involved with the treatment and care of the infected cases, have a higher exposure risk than others

➤ **Occupational contact dermatitis: It is the most common type of skin disease and is caused by** allergens, irritants, chemicals, temperatures, radiation, plants, animals, or parasites. Occupational contact dermatitis, or eczema, manifests as inflammation of the skin. Symptoms may include itching, pain, and redness as well as dry and flaky skin that can be easily treated and prevented.

➤ **Occupational Hearing Loss:** Hearing loss is a prevalent occupational disease due to the workplace. Loud noises and ototoxic chemicals are the main causes of occupational hearing loss. The symptoms can range from mild hearing loss to severe hearing loss. Prevention is the best treatment. The workers should not be exposed to noise exceeding 85Db for more than eight hours.

Prevention of Occupational Diseases: Common methods to prevent occupational diseases are

➤ Pre-placement examination

➤ Periodic examinations

➤ Medical and health care services

➤ Notifications

➤ Supervision of working environment

➤ Maintenance and analysis of records

➤ Health education and counselling

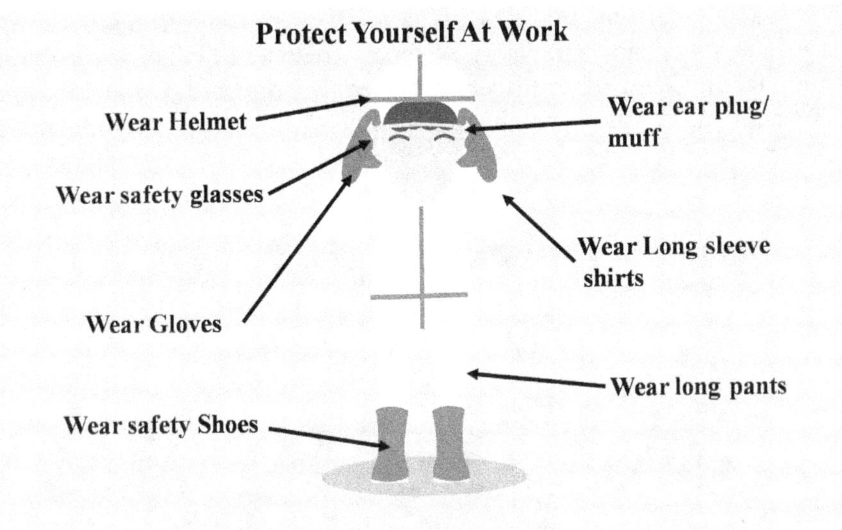

Figure 2.12 Prevention of occupational illnesses at work

Legislation: Recent regulations require most employers to adopt and enforce occupational health and safety programs to prevent the dangers of these diseases.

The National Policy on Safety, Health, and Environment at Workplace (NPSHEW)

> The National Policy on Safety, Health, and Environment at Workplace (NPSHEW) was declared by the Ministry of Labour & Employment, Govt of India, on 20th February 2009.

> The policy recognizes a safe and healthy working environment as a fundamental human right and aims to eliminate work-related injuries, diseases, etc,

> It aims to enhance the well-being of employees in all sectors of economic activity.

Solid Waste Disposal

The term solid waste usually includes

- **Garbage**: The term is given principally to food waste but may include other degradable organic wastes.
- **Rubbish**: consists of combustible and non-combustible solid waste, excluding food waste.
- **Refuse**: the collective term for solid waste includes both garbage and rubbish.
- **Litter:** bits of paper, discarded wrappings, bottles, left lying around in public places.

Solid waste refers to all types of garbage, trash, refuse, sludge from a wastewater treatment facility, water supply treatment facility, air pollution control facility, and other discarded materials originating from industrial, commercial, agricultural, and mining operations, as well as human activities.

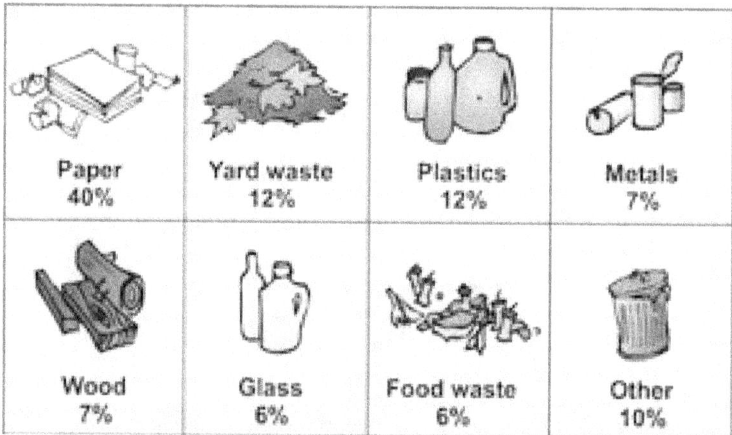

Figure 2.13 Various categories of municipal solid waste

Types of solid waste: Waste is generated continuously in every single way from our daily activities. Each activity will generate different types of waste which will require its own separate or specialized treatment. Solid waste is classified into different categories depending upon the source of origin:

(a) Municipal waste

(b) Industrial waste

(c) Biomedical or hospital solid waste

(d) Agricultural waste

Table 2.11 Different categories of solid waste

Category	Source of generation	Types of solid waste
Municipal solid waste	Residential (single and multi-family dwellings)	Food waste, rubbish, ashes, expired medicines
	Commercial (stores, hotels, markets, office buildings	Food waste, paper, cardboard, plastic, glass metal, Hazardous waste
	Open areas (parks, water bodies)	Rubbish
	Treatment plant sites	Treated waste, residual sludges
Industrial waste	Chemical industry, light, and heavy manufacturing, construction sites, oil refineries, fabrication, power and chemical plant	Hazardous materials, glass, asbestos. metals, scrap products, packaging, construction, and demolition material, housekeeping waste, waste from food processing, oil, solvents, paints, ceramics, stones, platic, rubber, leather, wood, cloth, straw

Table 2.11 *Contd...*

Category	Source of generation	Types of solid waste
Hazardous waste	Hospitals-biomedical waste	Hazardous by-products, petri dishes, surgical wraps, culture tubes, syringes, needles, blood vials, absorbent material, personal protective equipment, and pipette tips soiled waste, disposables, anatomical waste, cultures, discarded medicines, chemical wastes, etc., usually in the form of disposable syringes, swabs, bandages, body fluids, human excreta, etc
Agricultural waste	livestock waste, agricultural crop residues, and agro-industrial by-products	Residues generated from the production of rice (paddy husk), corn and wheat, rubber, coconut, etc. Pesticide organophosphate-herbicide-urea-fungicide-bearing waste.

Common ways of waste disposal:

Open dumping: It is an illegal process, in which any type of waste such as household trash, garbage, tires, demolition/construction waste, metal, or any other material dump at any location like along the roadside, vacant lots on public or private property even in parks other than approved landfill or facility. In underdeveloped countries, 60-90% of municipal solid waste is dumped in dangerous open dumps.

Landfills: It is the controlled disposal of waste on land in such a way that contact between waste and the environment is significantly reduced and the waste is concentrated in a well-defined area.

Challenges

Overflowing landfills: There is literally no space to accommodate huge garbage waste.

Degradation of waste: In nature, different categories of waste material decompose at different rates.

Table 2.12 Decomposition rates of different waste material

Biodegradable	Time to decompose (Years)	Non-biodegradable	Time to decompose (Years)
Paper role	2-4	Plastic foam	50
Disposable napkin	450	Plastic bag	10-20
Leather	50	Glass bottle	1 million
Banana peel	2-5	Nylon	30-40

Some alarming facts about the waste disposal problem in India are:

➢ Due to rapid population expansion, industry, monetary development, urbanization, and changed human lifestyles, the amount of municipal solid trash generated in India has increased.

➢ India produces 277.1 million tonnes of solid waste every year, which is likely to touch 387.8 million tonnes in 2030 and 543.3 million tons by 2050.

➢ 34 lakh tons of plastic waste was generated in 2019-20 which doubled in five years from 17 lakh tons in 2016. Covid added 8 million tons of plastic waste

➢ Increase in e-waste (TVs, computers, phones, etc.) to 10.14 lakh tons in 2020 from 7 .71 lakh tons 2019-20 with an increase of 31%

➢ Of the total collected waste, only 20 percent is processed and the remaining 80 percent is dumped in landfill sites that are turning into looming mountains of trash.

Effect on health and environment: The increasing volume of waste and its improper disposal is a serious matter of concern and is the main cause of all pollution i.e. air, water, and land, occupational. As a result of solid waste disposal, there are severe effects on human health and the environment:

➢ Uncollected solid waste can block storm water runoff, generating stagnant water bodies that breed disease-causing organisms

➢ Untreated waste thrown in rivers, seas, and lakes results in the accumulation of toxic substances in the food chain through the plants and animals that feed on it

➢ Plastic water bottles release a harmful component Diethylhydroxyl-amine (DEHA). (A carcinogen that affects reproduction, liver function, and weight loss.). DEHA leaks into soil and water, harming animal and plant life.

➢ Colored plastics are harmful as their pigment contains heavy metals like copper, lead, chromium cobalt, etc. that are highly toxic.

➢ Disposal of healthcare wastes can create major health hazards, such as Hepatitis B and C, through wounds caused by discarded syringes.

➢ Rag pickers who search at dumps for items that can be recycled may sustain injuries on coming in contact with hazardous items.

➢ Landfills are the major source of methane and other greenhouse gases

➢ The potential risks associated with municipal solid wastes to human health are:

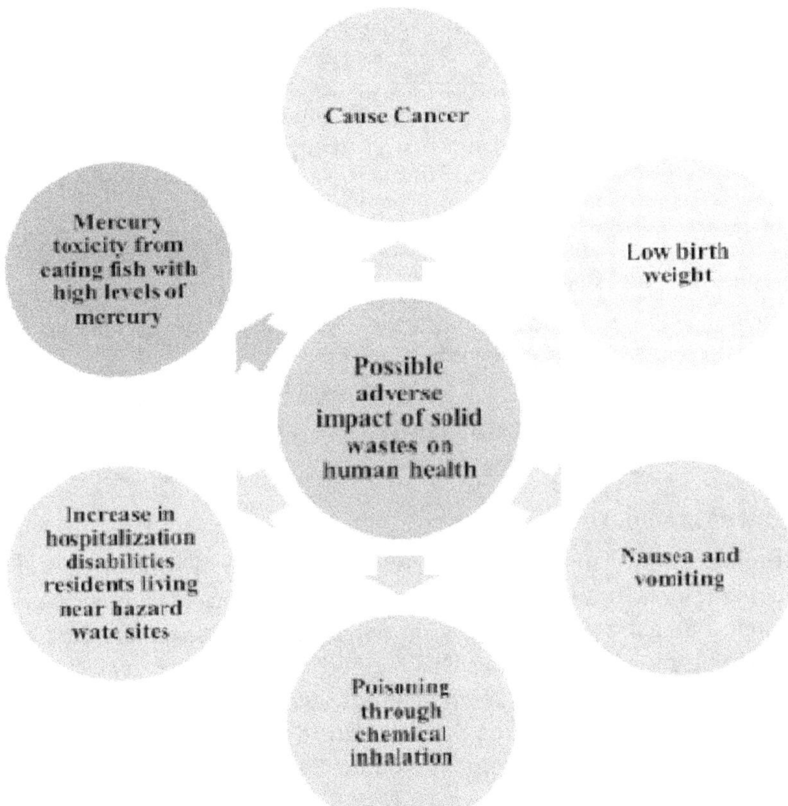

Figure 2.14 Risk associated with solid waste

Preventive measures: The excessive solid waste that is generated should be controlled by taking certain preventive measures. Integrated Solid Waste Management (ISWM) is a comprehensive waste collection, treatment, recovery, and disposal method that aims to provide environmental, sustainability, economic affordability, and social acceptance.

Collection methods:

Centralized method: The method involves the collection of municipal waste from all over the local area and disposing of it by means of the landfill, and dumping outside the City/Nagar panchayat limits. This process looks at a door-to-door collection of solid waste by waste pickers who hand it over to the collection team who then discard the collected waste in the landfill.

De-centralized method: The waste is collected and segregated at the source into bio-degradable and non-biodegradable. It improves collection efficiency and leads to better efficiency in the processing of waste.

Table 2.13 Segregation of waste

Colour coding	Type of container	Waste categories
Yellow	Plastic bag	Human anatomical waste/microbiological waste/items contaminated with blood and body fluids
Red	Disinfected container Plastic bag	Solid waste IV tubes/catheters
Blue/white translucent	Plastic bag/puncture-proof containers	Waste sharps/syringes/plastic tubes
Black	Plastic bags/puncture-proof containers	Discarded medicines/chemical waste/incineration ash

Treatment methods:

- **Incineration**: This method involves the burning of solid wastes at high temperatures until the wastes are turned into ashes. Incinerators are made in such a way that they do not give off extreme amounts of heat when burning solid wastes. This method of solid waste management can be done by individuals, municipalities, and even institutions. The good thing about this method is the fact that it reduces the volume of waste up to 20 or 30% of the original volume.

- **Pyrolysis:** Solid wastes are chemically decomposed by heat without the presence of oxygen. It usually occurs under pressure and at temperatures of up to 430°C. The solid wastes are changed into gasses, solid residue of carbon and ash, and small quantities of liquid.

- **Composting:** Due to a lack of adequate space for landfills, biodegradable waste is allowed to decompose It is a biological process in which micro-organisms, specifically fungi, and bacteria, convert degradable organic waste into substances like hummus. This finished product, which looks like soil, is high in carbon and nitrogen. Good quality environmentally friendly manure is formed from compost and can be used for agricultural purposes.

- **Waste disposal solutions**: The 4R Principle, which stands for reduce, reuse, recycle, and recover, is the most common solid waste management principle.

  - Reduce includes all the activities which reduce the generating of solid waste into the environment.

  - Reuse is the usage of any product itself without changing its form and composition.

> Recycle means re-covering a previously used object and giving it a second life.

> Recovery Most of the materials thrown in the garbage can be used & processed in ways other than being destroyed.

Sewage (Wastewater) Disposal

Sewage is the wastewater generated by a community, namely:

(a) Domestic wastewater, from bathrooms, toilets, kitchens, etc.,

(b) Raw or treated industrial wastewater   discharged into the sewerage system.

(c) Rainwater that has run down the street during a storm or heavy rain.

The sewage flow rate and composition vary from place to place, depending upon the economic aspects, social behavior, types of industries in the area, climatic conditions, water consumption and type of sewer system, etc.

Composition of Sewage

Sewage is a complex mixture containing suspended solids, organic and inorganic impurities, nutrients, saprophytes, and disease-causing bacteria and other microbes. These include the following

Table 2.14 Types of pollutants

Types of pollutants	Examples
Organic pollutants	Human feces, animal waste, urine
Inorganic pollutants	Nitrates, phosphates, metals
Nutrients	Phosphorus, nitrogen
Microorganisms	bacteria, virus, protozoans, helminthic
Chemicals	Heavy metals, trace metals, detergents, solvents, pesticides like pharmaceuticals, antibiotics, and hormones
Gases	H_2S, CH_4, NH_3, toxic compounds like oil from cars

Sewage disposal system: A system for disposing of sewage, industrial, or other wastes and includes sewage systems and treatment works. Manholes sewers, and sewerage make up the sewage system.

> **Sewers:** The pipes which carry wastewater.

> **Sewerage:** The network of sewers.

> **Manhole:** These are the holes made in sewers at frequent intervals so that timely inspections and cleaning of sewers can be done through them. The manhole is covered with a hard lid so that people and traffic can easily move over it.

Disposal methods: Following are 5 common methods of sewage disposal.

1. **Treatment plants:** Sewage treatment plants receive untreated sewage from municipal sewage systems. In multiple treatment sessions, the plants eliminate bacteria from the sewage.

2. **Sewage lagoons:** The home's wastewater flows into a pond of standing water. Wind and sunlight support the growth of beneficial microorganisms, resulting in natural sewage treatment.

3. **On-site systems**: In an on-site disposal system, wastewater is pumped into a septic tank, which collects the sludge and drains the water. Septic tanks must be pumped on a regular basis to prevent sludge accumulation.

4. **Off-site systems:** An off-site sewage system collects sewage from nearby homes and buildings and disinfects the water. The effluent is then sent to a community "water collection" before being dumped into a local water source (river, creek, etc.).

5. **Full sewage systems:** Solid waste from water is separated by blades fitted inside the pipes. The pipes then direct it to the treatment plant once everything has been minimized.

Challenges with wastewater:

➢ **Treatment of sewage**: The construction of toilets alone will not solve sanitation problems. While toilets are a part of the solution, a bigger issue is how to contain and treat India's sewage, as 93% of it ends out in ponds, lakes, and rivers without treatment.

➢ **Leaking and incomplete sewage systems**: raw sewage overflow, septic tanks, leaking sewer lines, land application of sludge, and partially treated wastewater contaminate rivers and lakes.

Nearly all sewage eventually makes its way into the aquatic ecosystem, where it contributes significantly to water contamination and constitutes a serious threat to human health. Examples of sewage-related pathogens and diseases they cause are included in the following table.

Table 2.15 Sewage-related pathogens and diseases

Pathogen class	Example	Disease
Bacterias	*Shigella sp., Salmonella sp.*	Dysentery Salmonellosis (gastroenteritis)
	Salmonella typhi	Typhoid fever
	Vibrio cholerae	Cholera
	Escherichia coli	
Viruses	*Hepatitis A virus*	Infectious hepatitis
	Rotaviruses	Acute gastroenteritis
	Polioviruses	Poliomyelitis

Table 2.15 contd....

Pathogen class	Example	Disease
Protozoas	*Entamoebahistolytica* *Giardia lamblia*	Amebiasis (amoebic dysentery) Giardiasis (gastroenteritis)
Helminths	*Ascaris sp.* *Taeniasp*	Ascariasis (roundworm infection) Taeniasis (tapeworm infection)

Methaemoglobinaemia: (also known as "blue-baby syndrome"), is a poisoning that can occur in infants during the first few months of life due to ingestion of well water high in nitrates. Improperly designed septic systems installed in sandy soils are known to cause nitrate contamination of groundwater.

Wastewater treatment plant (WWTP) or Sewage Treatment Plant: Effective sewage treatment is crucial for the economy, ecology, and public health since untreated wastewater can contaminate drinking water supplies and spread illness. Hence sewage is treated in sewage treatment plants (STPs) to make it less polluting. Treatment of wastewater involves physical, chemical, and biological processes, which remove physical, chemical and biological matter that contaminates the wastewater.

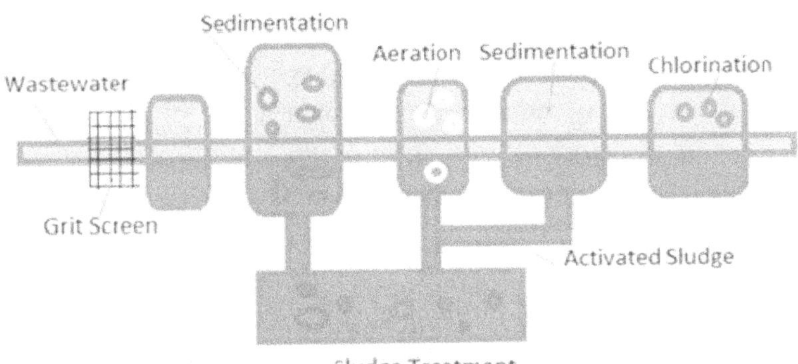

Figure 2.16 Working of sewage treatment plant

Physical Process:

1. **Filtration**: Wastewater is passed through bar screens. Large objects like rags, sticks, cans, plastic packets, and napkins removed.

2. **Grit and sand removal**: Water then goes to a grit and sand removal tank. The speed of the incoming wastewater is decreased to allow sand, grit, and pebbles to settle down.

3. **Sedimentation**: The water is then allowed to settle in a large tank which is sloped towards the middle. Solids like feces settle at the bottom and are removed with a scraper. This is the sludge. A skimmer removes the floatable solids like oil and grease. Water so cleared is

called clarified water. The sludge is transferred to a separate tank where it is decomposed by anaerobic bacteria. The biogas produced in the process can be used as fuel or can be used to produce electricity.

Biological Process: Aeration: Air is pumped into the clarified water to help aerobic bacteria to grow. Bacteria consume human waste, food waste, soaps, and other unwanted matter still remaining in clarified water.

Chemical process: Chlorination: Water purified through aeration is not fit for human consumption. It needs to be treated with chlorine. For this, bleaching powder is added to the water. Chlorine kills whatever germs may be left in the water. After chlorination, the water is fit for drinking.

Environmental Pollution due to Pharmaceuticals

➢ Pharmaceuticals are chemical compounds that are primarily utilized for medicinal and preventive purposes in both humans and animals.

➢ The pharmaceutical industry has provided numerous benefits in terms of protecting health but pharmaceuticals have also been identified as causing a global threat to environmental and human health.

➢ Biological pharmaceuticals such as vaccines, antibodies, insulin, vitamins, and other protein-based drugs are not considered environmental concerns because they are nearly always metabolized in humans and/or readily biodegradable. Non-biological pharmaceutical substances may end up in the environment.

Source of pharmaceutical pollution: The major sources identified for releasing pharmaceuticals and their metabolites into the environment are:

1. **Pharmaceutical industry:**

   ➢ Discharge from manufacturing units: The production facilities are an important source of environmental pollution. Wastewater treatment plants are unable to filter out chemical compounds used to manufacture drugs and personal care products, so these chemicals seep into freshwater systems and into the oceans.

   ➢ Emission of greenhouse gases: Through direct emission of greenhouse gases into the atmosphere from factories as a result of their production processes, and indirect through electricity use.

2. **Hospital waste:** Inappropriate management of drug-containing waste in hospitals

3. **Use of pharmaceuticals by patients:** Pharmaceuticals are excreted by patients in the same form or they are transformed by the body into metabolites, which may be released into the environment through sewers and sewage treatment plants.

Wastewater and sewage sludge from municipal wastewater treatment plants is the source of drugs excreted by humans not only in households but also in hospitals and other therapeutic facilities.

4. **Application of treated pharmaceutical waste in agriculture:** Widespread application of effluents and biosolids after wastewater treatment for fertilizing purposes contributes to the release of significant amounts of pharmaceuticals into the environment as some drugs are not degraded during treatment.

5. **Inappropriate disposal of unused or expired medicines**: Disposal of unused and expired medicines via solid household waste can also result in pharmaceutical residues entering the environment if this waste is dumped in landfills. Medicines discarded in sinks and flushed down in toilets enter sewage waters and, leak into aquatic systems.

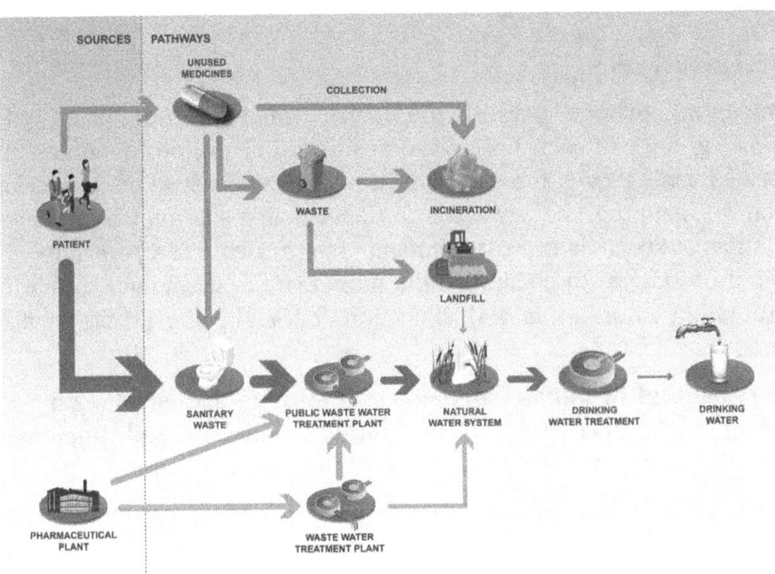

Figure 2.17 Main sources and pathways of pharmaceutical residues in the environment

Effects of Pharmaceutical Pollution: Some of the major threats are:

➢ Pollution of water-related ecosystems directly threatens people's health and livelihoods, and affects the economy of the country.

➢ **Risk to aquatic life:** Pharmaceutical contaminants result in the depletion of oxygen and pose risk to aquatic and human life forms in the river by entering the food chain.

➢ **Antimicrobial resistance (AMR):** Antimicrobial resistance is the single greatest threat to humanity. AMR occurs when bacteria, fungi, viruses, and parasites evolve resistance to common antibiotics, making them ineffective. For example, once-curable infections like tuberculosis are harder to fight off, or even impossible because of multi-drug-resistant tuberculosis.

Main causes of AMR

➢ During the manufacture of antibiotics, residual material and ingredients can seep into the water, which is then discharged into the surrounding environment. This can contribute to the emergence and spread of AMR.

➢ Over-prescribing and inappropriate use of antibiotics by humans, as well as improper disposal.

➢ Use of antibiotics in intensive livestock farming, e.g., to promote growth and prevent infection.

➢ Release of AMR-contributing compounds into the environment from manufacturing sites.

Control Measures

Encouraging proper use of medicines: Medicines are not ordinary consumer goods. At each link in the healthcare chain, professionals, public authorities, patients and the public must be informed about the proper use of medicines. Inappropriate use leads to unnecessary and avoidable emissions of pharmaceuticals in the environment. Pharmaceutical companies should engage in initiatives to encourage the proper use of medicines, in particular by promoting information and education for healthcare professionals and patients.

Proper disposal of unused medicines: Informing and encouraging people regarding the proper disposal of unused medicines and implementing systems that collect and properly dispose of unused medicines.

The responsible use of antibiotics: The 5 key to reducing antibiotic concentrations is the responsible prescription and use of antibiotics and investing in new technologies to improve the efficiency of wastewater treatment plants (WWTP).

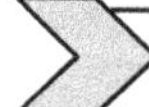

2.5 Psychosocial Pharmacy

➢ Drug misuse, drug abuse, drug dependence, and drug addiction are important social health problems that are widespread and affect a large population.

➢ This health problem is also termed a substance abuse disorder. Substance abuse is the dangerous or addictive use of psychoactive compounds i.e. chemical that affects brain activity "mood-altering" drug.

➤ Psychoactive drugs: These are addictive, typically depressing or exciting, or alter perception. Its social relevance is presumed to be very high as it predominantly alters the psychosocial health (**social behavior**) of a person.

Medicines:

1. **Medicines** are legal drugs that help the body to recover from an injury, infection, illness, or disease.

2. **An over-the-counter** drug is a medication that can be purchased legally in pharmacies and other retailers without a doctor's prescription. If the recommendations on the label are not followed, such medications may be harmful.

3. A **prescription drug** is a chemical substance that may only be obtained/purchased with a valid prescription from a doctor.

4. An **illegal drug** is a chemical substance that people of any age may not lawfully manufacture, possess, buy, or sell.

Drug Misuse

Drug misuse is not a disorder. It is generally related to prescription medicines. It refers to the incorrect use of prescription or over-the-counter medicines. If the instructions are not followed, these medications can have negative effects. Repeated drug misuse can lead to drug abuse and eventually addiction e.g.

➤ Taking more of a prescription than is prescribed.

➤ Taking drugs with the wrong meals or at the wrong time of the day.

➤ Misusing medication for an extended period of time.

➤ Taking medicine for purposes other than those prescribed.

➤ Taking a drug that was not prescribed to you

Drug Abuse

➤ Drug abuse occurs when any drug is used improperly or used unsafely for non-therapeutic purposes.

➤ Drug abuse occurs when drugs, such as alcohol, illegal narcotics, or psychotropic substances, are misused to seek pleasure or create self-harm. Drug abuse impacts one's thoughts, behavior, and body functioning.

➤ The key difference between a person who misuses drugs and a person who abuses drugs is their intent. The former takes a drug to treat a specific disease condition, whereas the latter uses a drug to generate certain feelings.

Why drugs are misused or abused?

➢ Many psychoactive drugs trigger activity along a pathway of cells in the brain called the **"reward pathway."**

➢ Brain cells along the activated reward pathway release a chemical called dopamine.

➢ Dopamine is a neurotransmitter that is released during a pleasurable experience. Substance use leads to the release of such neurotransmitters, including dopamine, associated with the reward circuit in the brain. The continued release of dopamine associated with a pleasurable experience leads to changes in the brain leading to dependence. Activities associated with the pleasurable experience can trigger cravings even after substance use is stopped.

➢ The extra dopamine released during drug use can cause the user to ignore the harmful effects of the drug and want to continue using it.

➢ Flooding the reward pathway with dopamine may lead to intense cravings for the drug.

➢ After a time, drug abuse can dull the brain's reactions to natural levels of dopamine.

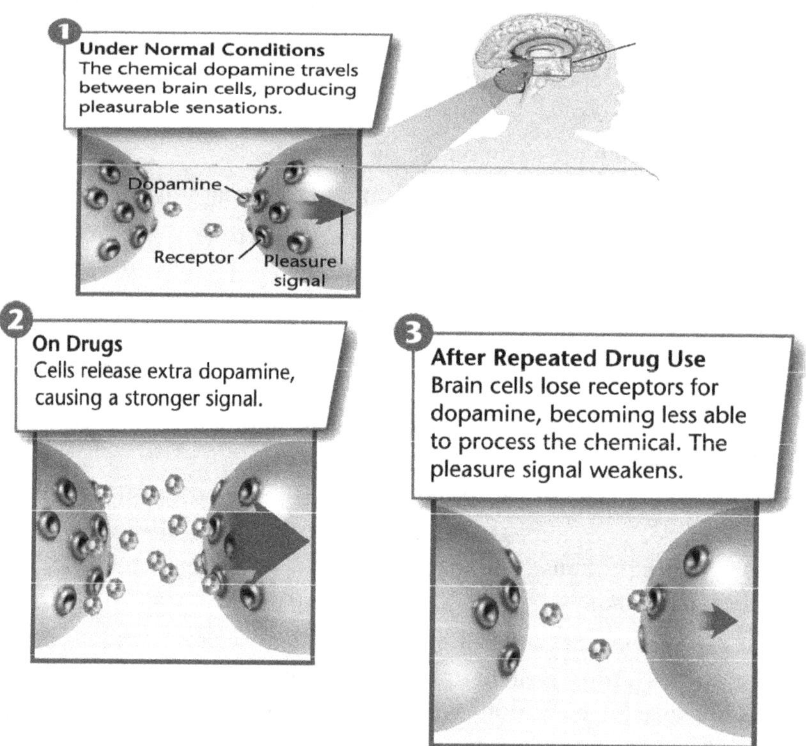

Figure 2.18 Pathway of psychoactive drugs

Drugs of abuse may be classified into:

- ➤ **Permissive drugs:** The usage of these drugs is commonly accepted as a social norm. Caffeine is a stimulant in tea, coffee, and cola drinks, nicotine in the form of cigarette smoking, gutkha/khaini, and alcohol drinking at social gatherings.

- ➤ **Prescriptive medications** are used therapeutically to treat specific diseases and are available only with a doctor's prescription. The same drugs can be abused by vulnerable people. Sedatives, hypnotics, and amphetamines.

- ➤ **Proscriptive drugs:** This category includes those drugs which have been placed under strict drug control to avoid their illicit or illegal use. Some medically used drugs, such as opioid stimulants, fall into this category when used for non-medical purposes. The majority of abused medicines are psychoactive.

Dangers of drug misuse and abuse: Misusing or abusing medications can have major health consequences. When a person uses a drug repeatedly, the body may develop tolerance to the drug. Tolerance may lead to drug dependence.

- ➤ **Drug dependence** is defined as a circumstance or state in which a person uses or abuses a drug to the point where it becomes the main focus of his life. Taking a drug becomes a compulsion, a required habit.

- ➤ **Physical Dependence:** Long-term use in large levels changes body chemistry. The person becomes habitual.

- ➤ **Psychological Dependence**: The abuser is using drugs because he believes he needs them which is more of a mental or emotional need.

- ➤ **Addiction:** Addiction is excessive drug usage. It affects the structure and chemistry of the brain, resulting in the inability to stop using a substance regardless of the cost to health, family, or social standing.

People with drug addiction have a physical and/or psychological dependence on a particular substance. If such a person stops taking the drug, then the person will experience severe **withdrawal symptoms.** Withdrawal symptoms include nausea or vomiting, headaches or dizziness, digestion problems, fever, paranoia or panic, tremors, seizures, or death.

When a drug does more to you than for you and yet you continue to use it, it is termed addiction.

Following are a few drugs that have addictive potential:

1. **Tobacco Products:** Nicotine is a harmful chemical obtained from Nicotiana tobacco that causes drug dependence. It is used in cigars, cigarettes, beedi, hooka, snuff, jarda, khaini, gutka, etc. When nicotine is

inhaled as smoke, it is quickly absorbed. One cigarette raises plasma nicotine by 15 to 30 mg/ml in 10 minutes.

Tobacco Addiction:

- Excess intake of nicotine causes adverse effects like seizures, coma, and even death due to respiratory. Chronic smokers have a high risk of cancer attacks. Thrombosis induced by smoking results in coronary heart disease.

- Nicotine withdrawal causes cigarette cravings. Symptoms last for a month. Other symptoms are anxiety, insomnia, restlessness, etc.

Treatment of Nicotine dependence and withdrawal symptoms: *Nicotine Replacement Therapy* is found useful in treating nicotine dependence where a substitute to nicotine is administered to the dependents who contain relatively small amounts of nicotine. Other drugs like Bupropion, Rimonabant, Varenicline, and Clonidine are also used.

2. **Alcohol:**

- Alcohol abuse is a common problem. Since alcohol is heavily marketed, and commonly available, many people suffer from alcoholism.

- Alcohol depresses the CNS. Alcohol affects behavior. Driving judgment and coordination are compromised at low doses.

- Low to moderate doses of alcohol might leads to the likelihood of many aggressive behaviors, such as the abuse of partners and children.

- Moderate to high doses of alcohol significantly impairs brain functioning altering a person's ability to learn and remember information.

- Very high doses cause respiratory depression and death.

- Continued use of alcohol can lead to dependence.

- Sudden discontinuation of alcohol intake is likely to produce withdrawal symptoms, including severe anxiety, tremors, hallucinations, and convulsions.

Alcohol addiction

- Alcohol elevates dopamine, 5-HT, acetylcholine, and norepinephrine and enhances drug dependence activity since it produces pleasant feelings.

- Chronic alcohol consumption produces various adaptive neuronal changes

- Alcohol consumption is associated with adverse consequences in all aspects of life, including social, legal, occupational, psychological, and medical issues.

> Withdrawal symptoms such as anxiety and tremor develop after a short period without a drink and are reduced by taking more alcohol. Generally, alcohol dependence remains undetected for years.

Treatment of alcoholism:

> Aversion therapy is a common treatment for alcoholism.

> Disulfiram is a popular therapeutic medicine, but it comes with its own set of side effects.

> Sedatives and hypnotics, such as chlordiazepoxide and diazepam, ease withdrawal symptoms to some extent, preventing seizures, delirium, and arrhythmias.

> Giving glucose, thiamine, and other electrolytes helps to cure alcohol poisoning by minimizing respiratory depression.

> Acamprosate is another drug of choice for alcoholics.

> Naltrexone, an opioid receptor antagonist, can help addicts reduce their alcohol cravings.

3. **Narcotics:**

> Narcotics refer to opium, opium derivatives, and their semi-synthetic substitutes,

> The two most common forms of narcotic drugs are morphine and codeine. Both are synthesized from opium for medicinal purposes.

> An opioid is any psychoactive chemical that resembles morphine in its pharmacological effects.

> Commonly abused opioids are morphine, heroin, codeine, oxycodeine, meperidine.

Addiction with Narcotics:

> Opioids alter brain chemistry and lead to drug tolerance. Long-term opioid use results in withdrawal symptoms (such as muscle cramping, diarrhea, and anxiety). All long-term opiate users become dependent, though few become addicted.

> Psychological dependence on narcotics is characterized by craving. The increased dopamine levels enhance the craving effect. The symptoms of physical dependence include GI upset, mydriasis, cough, hyperventilation, ocular discharge, diarrhea, yawning, hyperthermia, aggressiveness, and vomiting.

> Sudden withdrawal effects are termed noradrenergic storms due to the increased release of norepinephrine.

Treatment of opioid dependence:

1. Lofexidine, an α-2-adrenergic receptor agonist is also effective against the withdrawal effects of opioids.
2. Opioid agonist like Naltrexone is effective against euphoria and withdrawal symptoms of opioids.
3. Replacement therapy with Methadone, and buprenorphine. is found useful in treating opioid dependence.

4. Psychotropics

➤ Most psychoactive medications have strict prescription guidelines and can only be supplied with a valid prescription, yet these drugs are abused.

➤ Psychotropic drugs affect behavior, mood, thinking, and perception. They change normal levels of dopamine, GABA, norepinephrine, and serotonin and build dependency. Various prescription drugs are abused e.g.

- **Dependence on sedatives and hypnotics:** If the barbiturate is used regularly for more than a month, the brain develops a demand for it, which results in severe symptoms. If the drug is stopped tremors, difficulty in sleeping, and irritability are all signs of withdrawal.

- **Dependence on antianxiety drugs:** The prolonged use of benzodiazepine drugs causes it. It is characterized by a withdrawal syndrome in response to a drop-in benzodiazepine blood plasma levels after dose reduction or abrupt withdrawal. Tolerance to the sleep-inducing effects of benzodiazepines develops quickly.

- **Dependence on antidepressants:** Misusing imipramine can be harmful, like other drugs. Long-term use of large doses of imipramine may make it difficult to stop. The medicine makes people crave it when they don't need it, which is harmful. Long-term use decreases the medicine's effectiveness.

Effects of substance use disorders on family: The effects of Substance Use Disorders on the family may include:

➤ **Emotional burden:** Anxiety, anger, frustration, fear, concern, despair, humiliation and guilt, or embarrassment may be experienced by family members.

➤ **Financial burden:** This could be the result of drug use, job loss.

➤ **Dissatisfaction in relationships:** Families may face significant levels of tension and conflict as a result of substance use.

- **Family breakdown**: Abuse or violence can lead to a family breakup.
- **Effects on the developing fetus and children:** Alcohol consumption during pregnancy can cause birth abnormalities and developmental difficulties in offspring. Cognitive impairment is more common among babies delivered to opioid-dependent mothers. Children of parents with SUDs are at increased risk for abuse or neglect.
- **Effects on parents:** Mothers with SUDs are less sensitive and less emotionally available to infants.

Social effects of substance use disorders: SUDs have an impact on people's social functioning and impose a burden on society. The issues linked with SUD are:

- Housing insecurity, homelessness, and criminal activity.
- HIV transmission through IV drug use or high-risk sexual activities.
- Unemployment or welfare dependency is also a societal issue linked to SUDs.
- Physical and psychological disorders, disability.
- Due to the high cost of treating addiction, medical, and psychiatric diseases, these social issues place a financial strain on society and governments.

CHAPTER 3

Nutrition and Health

Food is a basic requirement of life. It can be anything solid or liquid that provides energy in the form of calories, aids in the growth of new cells, repairs old and worn-out cells and tissues, provides immunity for fighting various infectious diseases, and keeps the body in balance by regulating and controlling various functions when swallowed, digested, and assimilated in the body. Good nutrition is consuming nutrient-dense meals that meet the body's nutritional requirements, allowing it to grow and stay healthy.

Nutrition is the science of food/nutrients and their relationship to health and sickness.

LEARNING OBJECTIVES

- Basics of nutrition – Macronutrients and micronutrients, Importance of water and fibers in the diet
- Balanced diet, malnutrition, nutrition deficiency diseases, ill effects of junk foods, calorific and nutritive values of various foods, fortification of food
- Introduction to food safety, adulteration of foods, effects of artificial ripening, use of pesticides, genetically modified foods
- Dietary supplements, nutraceuticals, food supplements – indications, benefits, Drug-Food Interactions

3.1 Basics of Nutrition

Nutrients

Nutrients are dietary components that must be provided in sufficient amounts to the body. The major are carbohydrates, proteins, lipids, minerals, vitamins, water, and fibers.

Classification of Nutrients: Nutrients can be classified as macronutrients and micronutrients on the basis of the required quantity to be consumed every day.

1. **Macronutrients:** (Macro means huge): The body needs enormous amounts of certain nutrients to function properly, such as proteins, carbohydrates, lipids, and fibers.

2. **Micronutrients:** (Needed in modest quantities) Vitamins and minerals.

1. Macronutrients

(i) Carbohydrates:

Carbohydrate is the most important component of the diet. Its main objective is to provide the body with energy in the form of calories. The three primary sources of carbohydrates are starches, sugars, and cellulose.

Food sources for carbohydrates: wheat, bajra, rice, jowar, jaggery, honey, and some fruits

Important functions:

> Carbohydrates are an important energy source. Each gram of carbohydrate provides 4 kilocalories. These are absorbed as glucose by the body. Glucose conducts a series of metabolic processes in order to produce ATPs (adenosine triphosphate), the cell's energy currency.

> Surplus glucose is stored as glycogen (glycogenesis) in the liver and skeletal muscles after the body's needs have been met. Glycogen reserves can be used during sleeping, fasting, or following a calorie-restricted diet.

(ii) Proteins:

The term "protein" comes from the Greek word protos, which means "first". Protein is the most fundamental chemical unit in living creatures, and it is required for nourishment, the formation of new tissues (growth), and the maintenance and repair of those that have already been formed.

Food sources: casein from milk, albumin from eggs, and gluten from wheat.

Important Functions:

> Proteins are required for growth, body construction, as well as tissue repair, and maintenance.

> Proteins make up the majority of enzymes engaged in numerous chemical processes that occur within the body.

> Proteins make up some of the most vital hormones, such as glucagon and insulin.

> Collagen is a protein that provides bones, teeth, and skin structure, whereas keratin is a protein found in hair and nails.

> Some proteins, such as immunoglobulins, are antibodies that play a key role in immunity.

> Proteins regulate osmotic pressure. If protein intake is insufficient to maintain normal blood protein levels, fluid will enter the surrounding tissues and cause edema (swelling).

- ➢ Proteins are responsible for transporting nutrients and other chemicals e.g. hemoglobin, which transports oxygen.
- ➢ Proteins help to maintain acid-base balance and a neutral pH by acting as buffers.
- ➢ Protein serves as an energy reserve. Though the body does not rely on proteins to meet its energy needs, protein from the muscles and other tissues is used as an energy source after extended fasting or low carbohydrate consumption

(iii) Fats:

Lipids or dietary fats are high-energy foods, with each gram giving up to 9 kcal. Fats in meals include oils found in seeds, butter from milk, and lard from pork. The final products of fat digestion include fatty acids and glycerol. Most fatty acids are made in the body, with the exception of linoleic acid (LA) and alpha-linolenic acid (ALA), and must be received from food.

Food sources: Visible fat sources are butter, lard, ghee oils, and eggs while invisible fat sources are cereals, pulses, oil seeds,

Linoleic acid: Sunflower oil, Corn oil, Soya bean oil, Sesame oil, Groundnut oil Mustard oil Palm oil Coconut oil.

Alpha-Linolenic acid: Soya bean oil, Leafy greens

Important functions:

- ➢ Fats act as an **energy reserve** and can provide 9 kcal/gram. The use of fat-derived energy will spare proteins for tissue growth and repair.
- ➢ Dietary fats dissolve and transport fat-soluble vitamins such as vitamins A, D, E, and K, and also disease-fighting phytochemicals like carotenoids.
- ➢ Diet rich in fat may provide **essential fatty acids** necessary for growth and other important functions.
- ➢ Give satiety.
- ➢ Fats deposited in adipose tissues act as **insulators** against heat and cold.
- ➢ Fats in the body support viscera such as the heart, kidneys, intestine, and other vital organs.

2. Micronutrients

Minerals

(i)   Calcium:

Calcium is present in both animal and plant foods. The richest source of calcium among animal foods is milk, green leafy vegetables like amaranth, fenugreek, drumstick, ragi, dry nuts, and certain oil seeds.

Important Functions: Calcium serves a variety of functions in humans, including:

➢ Calcium is essential for growth since it is a component of bones and teeth, as well as the regular functioning of all cells in the body.

➢ Calcium is required for the formation of blood clots.

➢ Calcium is required for the contraction of many muscles, including cardiac, skeletal, and smooth muscles, in order for them to function effectively.

Calcium deficiency: Calcium deficiency can lead to osteoporosis (a loss of bone density and mass), osteomalacia (a loss of bone quality), osteopenia (poor bone density), and tetany (a tingling sensation in the hands and feet).

(ii) Phosphorus:

Phosphorus is a necessary mineral for the normal functioning of every cell in the body. Phosphorus is present in the body as phosphate (PO_4^{3-}). Around 85% of the phosphorous in the body is found in bones and teeth whereas 15% of soft tissues contain it. High blood phosphorus levels have been related to an increased risk of cardiovascular diseases.

Food sources: Milk, beef, whole grain cereals, legumes, almonds, carrots, and shellfish are all high in phosphorus.

Important functions:

➢ It assists in the formation of bones and teeth, together with calcium and magnesium. It also helps to make phospholipids, which are important components of cell structure.

➢ DNA and RNA (nucleic acids) require phosphorus to function.

➢ Phosphorylated substances such as adenosine triphosphate (ATP) and creatine phosphate are used in all kinds of energy synthesis and storage.

➢ The activation of numerous enzymes, hormones, and cell signaling requires phosphorylation.

➢ Phosphorus is also important for maintaining a healthy acid-base balance (pH).

➢ 2,3-diphosphoglycerate (2,3-DPG), a phosphorus-containing molecule, controls oxygen delivery to the body via hemoglobin.

Deficiency: Because phosphorus is so widely distributed in foods, dietary phosphorus deficiency requires near total starvation.

(iii) Iron:

➢ About 60 percent of iron in the body is found in hemoglobin, 5% in myoglobin, 5% in enzymes, and the remaining 30% in iron storing proteins ferritin and hemosiderin. Hemoglobin is the protein in red blood cells responsible for carrying oxygen to the tissues from the lungs. Myoglobin is a protein found in muscles and used for the storage of oxygen.

➢ Some foods affect the absorption of iron in the body e.g. Ascorbic acid increases and calcium, phytates decrease its absorption.

➢ Iron can be found in cereals, millets, pulses, and green leafy vegetables. Both bajra and ragi are high-iron cereal grains and millets. Plant foods include rice flakes, mint, soya beans, and dates. Animal sources of food include red meat and fish like mackerel.

Important Functions:

➢ It is a component of cell enzyme systems that oxidize glucose and other energy-producing substances.

➢ It plays a key part in the creation of immune cells that fight foreign microorganisms entering the body.

➢ Iron is required for proper brain development, neurotransmitter production, and breakdown.

➢ Hemoglobin has about 3.34 mg of iron per gram and is involved in transporting and storing oxygen.

Iron deficiency: The common causes are decreased iron in the diet, poor absorption of iron from the gut, acute and chronic blood loss, and increased demand for iron in certain situations like pregnancy or recovery from trauma or surgery. The decreased iron in the hemoglobin causes anemia. There are 3 types of anemia depending upon the size of the RBC:

➢ Microcytic: size of the RBC is less than normal

➢ Normocytic: size normal but less in number

➢ Macrocytic: larger than normal

Anemia may be avoided by eating iron-rich meals, vitamin C-rich foods, and seasonal fruits and vegetables on a regular basis.

(iv) Iodine:

It is one of the essential micronutrients for the healthy growth and development of the human body and brain. The human body contains iodine in levels of 15-20 mg. Iodine is an important component of the thyroid hormone, thyroxine.

Sources of Iodine: Iodine is abundant in marine fish and eggs. The iodization of salt is still the most cost-effective method of delivering iodine to humans and cattle, and it is credited for eliminating the iodine shortage.

Important Functions of Iodine: Iodine though required in small quantities is needed to perform the following functions

➤ Required for the synthesis of the thyroid hormone thyroxine (T4) and triiodothyronine (T3) which governs growth, development, reproduction, and basal metabolic rate.

➤ Thyroid hormones are able to control the conversion of carotene to active vitamin A.

Iodine deficiency: Deficiency of iodine causes

➤ Goiter: Goiter is a swelling of the thyroid gland caused by a lack of iodine in adequate levels to generate a normal amount of thyroxine.

➤ Cretinism: It is a congenital condition marked by physical deformities, dwarfism, and mental retardation, and is commonly due to a lack of iodine and thyroxin production.

(v) Zinc:

Zinc is the most essential trace element found within cells. An adult human carries 2g of zinc, 60% of which is found in skeletal muscle and 30% in bones.

Food sources: Meat, seafood, and liver are good sources of Zinc. In cereals, most of the zinc is found in the outer fiber-rich part of the kernel.

Important Functions of Zinc: The functions of zinc include:

➤ Important components in the creation of DNA, building proteins.

➤ Helps in digestion and metabolism.

➤ Controls the function of the male prostate.

Zinc deficiency: Growth retardation, dermatitis, hair loss, diarrhea, increased infections, delayed wound healing, loss of appetite, hypogeusia (diminished taste), dysgeusia (altered flavor), are some of the clinical signs of severe zinc deficiency in humans. Zinc deficiency can cause low birth weight and premature delivery.

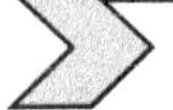

3.2   Importance of Water and Fibres in Diet

Water

Water is the main and the most significant component of the human body. The body cannot produce enough water through metabolism to meet its demands. As a result, we must ensure that we get enough water to meet our daily needs. Failing to do so could be harmful to our health. The most frequent symptoms are headaches, exhaustion, constipation, heat exhaustion, and reduced brain function.

Water accounts for about 70 percent of lean body mass. In adults, about two-thirds of total water is in the intracellular spaces, whereas one-third is extracellular water. A 70-kg human has about 42 L of total body water, of which 28 L is intracellular water and 14 L is extracellular fluid (ECF), of the latter, 3 L is in blood plasma, 1 L is the transcellular fluid (cerebrospinal fluid, ocular, pleural, peritoneal and synovial fluids) and 10 L is the interstitial fluid, including lymph, which provides an aqueous medium surrounding cell.

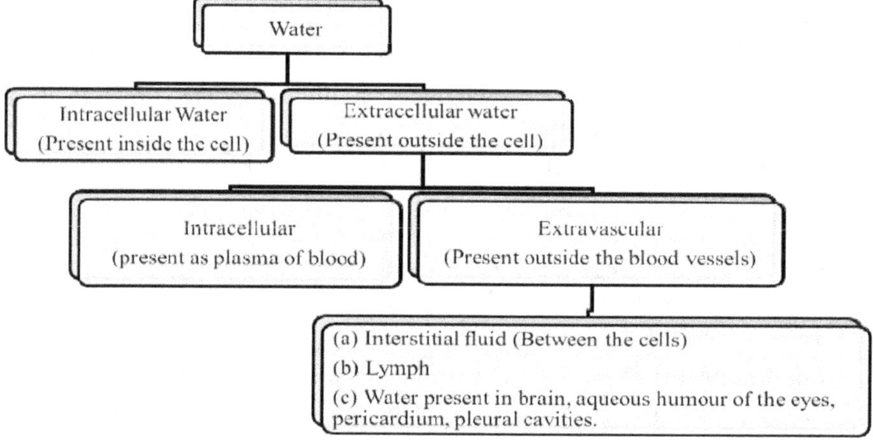

Figure 3.1 Distribution of water in the body

Role of water

Water has numerous roles and is needed for most body functions:
- Maintains the health and integrity of every cell in the body.
- Keeps the blood liquid enough to flow through blood vessels.
- Helps to eliminate the by-products of the body's metabolism, excess electrolytes (Sodium & Potassium), and urea, which is a waste product formed through the processing of dietary proteins.
- Regulates body temperature through sweating.
- Moistens mucous membranes (such as those of the lungs and mouth).
- Lubricates and cushions joints.
- Reduces the risk of urinary tract infections by keeping the bladder clear of bacteria.
- It aids in digestion and prevents constipation.
- Moisturises the skin to maintain its texture and appearance.
- Carry nutrients and oxygen to cells.
- Serves as a shock absorber inside the eyes, spinal cord, and in the amniotic sac surrounding the foetus in pregnancy.

Dietary Sources of water: Water must be consumed throughout the day because it is constantly lost through breath, perspiration, urine, and bowel movements. Water can be replenished in the body through water-rich fruits and vegetables in addition to consuming fluids e.g.

Table 3.1 Food sources of water

Food	Water content	Source
Cucumber	96%	Vitamins and fibres
Tomatoes	95%	Vitamin A
Spinach	93%	Iron
Mushrooms	92%	Vitamin B2
Orange	86%	VitC,fibres,antioxidants
Brocolli	90%	VitK,A,iron,Folic acid
Apple	86%	Fibre
Melon	91%	Potassium

Benefits of Water-Rich Foods

- Water-rich foods also function as detox agents, which help in cleansing the body of the accumulated toxins through various metabolic processes.
- Foods low in water, mainly protein and fat-rich foods like meat and meat products, cheese, nuts, and oilseeds, etc. require high amounts of water to be metabolized and excreted which can be done effectively by incorporating fruits and vegetables into the diet.
- Foods high in water also help in preventing fatigue and exhaustion because they are high in fructose and fibre, both of which serve to keep blood sugar levels normal.

Dietary Fibres

Dietary fibres known as roughage or bulk, are one of the most important components of the diet since it aids in digestion and nutritional absorption.

Dietary fibres are plant components that our bodies cannot digest or absorb, while lipids, proteins, and carbohydrates are easily absorbed and digested. The fibres remain unchanged as they pass through the stomach, small intestine, and colon before leaving our bodies.

The ICMR (Indian Council of Medical Research) advises 40 g of dietary fibre per day.

Classification of Dietary Fibres: Dietary fibres are commonly classified as soluble, which dissolve in water and forms a gel-like substance, or insoluble, which doesn't dissolve.

- ➢ **Food rich in soluble dietary fibres:** fruit, oats, beans and barley.
- ➢ **Food rich in insoluble dietary fibers:** wholemeal bread, wheat bran, vegetables and nuts.

Functions of soluble dietary fibre: Soluble fibres help to:

➤ Slow food passage through the stomach and into the small intestine. This prevents glucose absorption into the bloodstream, allowing one to feel fuller for extended periods of time. It aids in the management of blood sugar levels in diabetic people.

➤ Support the growth of friendly bacteria needed to help maintain a healthy gut.

➤ Reduce cholesterol absorption by binding to it in the gut. So lowers blood cholesterol levels.

Functions of insoluble dietary fibre: Theses kind of fibres add bulk to stools by absorbing water, and help to prevent constipation. It is important to increase your fluid intake along with a high fibre diet. Without fluid, the fibres stay hard, making it difficult to pass and may cause constipation.

Table 3.2 Health benefits of fibres

Health Benefits		
1.	**Digestive Health**	**Normalises** bowel movement **Bulk-up** make them easier to pass **Prevent** Constipation and diarrhoea
2.	**Diabetes**	**Improve** blood sugar level
3.	**Heart Health**	**Reduce** cardiac risk by decreasing LDL
4.	**Weight loss**	**Maintain** healthy weight

3.3   Balanced Diet

The term "balanced diet" refers to a diet consisting of a variety of foods in specific quantities and proportions that give adequate amounts of the nutrients required for good health.

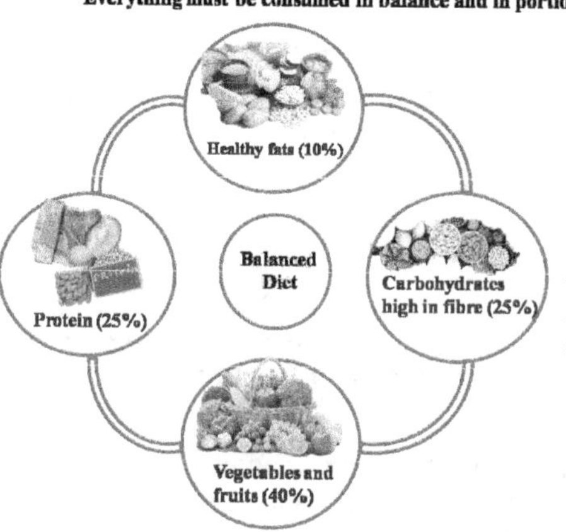

Figure 3.2 Balanced Diet

Components of a Balanced Diet

There are four key essential nutrients that make up a balanced diet:

➤ Fruits and vegetables (40%),

➤ Proteins (25%)

➤ Fibre-rich carbohydrates (25%)

➤ Good fats (10%)

Fruits and vegetables: They are the essential components of a balanced diet, and variety is as important as quantity. Vegetables can be classified into:

➤ **Leafy green vegetables:** contain the unique component chlorophyll. Greens are a treasure of nutrients like calcium, magnesium, potassium, omega-3 fatty acids, vitamins, and minerals.

➤ **Carotenoid (colored) vegetables**: They are a rich source of fibre and have antioxidant properties.

Fruits: Fruits give an adequate supply of vitamins, minerals, potassium, folates antioxidants

Importance: A diet rich in vegetables and fruits can help in:

➤ Lowering blood pressure and reducing the risk of heart disease.

➤ Prevent some types of cancer.

➤ Lower risk of eye and digestive problems.

➤ Positive effect on blood sugar.

➤ Promote weight loss: non-starchy vegetables and fruits like apples, pears, and green leafy vegetables promote weight loss.

➤ Fruits and vegetables are low in fat, salt, and sugar and a good source of dietary fibre.

➤ Balance the body's pH levels and control acidity e.g. cucumber, bottle gourd, spinach.

Daily fruit intake: 5 different types of vegetables and two fruits

Table 3.3 Interesting Facts of fruits and vegetables

Red Food	Contains Lycopene, helps in fighting cancer
White Food	Contains Sulphoraphan, anticancer
Blue Food	Contains anthocynins acts as antioxidants
Green Food	Contains unique components chlorophyll, spinach contains Lutein, Kale-Zeaxanthin (For old diseases)
Citrus Fruits	Vitamin C-only vitamin which the body cannot synthesize Promote the body's production of collagen, an important anti-aging component

Proteins: It is the second most abundant substance in the body after water. On average, 43 % of the protein in the body is found in the muscle, with considerable proportions being present in the skin (15%) and blood (16 %). The primary protein types in the body include collagen (connective tissue), haemoglobin, myosin, and actin (muscle fibres). Our protein needs change as we age and this is particularly true during childhood, adolescence, and pregnancy. Proteins can be extracted from many different sources:

A. Plant sources

a)   Soy products: Tofu (bean curd) and soybeans.

b)   Legume flours: Chickpea flour (Besan), lentil flour, and soy flour.

c)   Dried beans and peas: Red kidney beans (Rajmah), chickpeas and lentils (pulses).

d)   Dairy products: Milk, Cheese, Curd.

B. Animal sources

Eggs, lean meat, chicken, fish,

Functions: The major functions of proteins:

➤ **Build:** Protein is an integral part of bones, muscles, cartilage, and skin; for example, hair and nails are primarily composed of protein.

➤ **Repair:** It is used by the body to create and repair tissues.

➤ **Oxygenate.** Red blood cells are composed of a protein that transports oxygen throughout the body. This helps provide the entire body with the necessary nutrients.

➤ **Digest.** About half of the daily protein ingested is used to produce enzymes, which aid in digestion, as well as to generate new cells and body chemicals.

➤ **Regulate:** Protein has an important feature role in the regulation of hormones.

Carbohydrates: Carbohydrates are the main fuel for the brain and muscles. 60 % of the daily calories come from carbohydrates. The body breaks down carbohydrates into glucose which flows through the blood to cells with the help of insulin. Carbohydrates are the main source of energy for the cell to function.

Sources: The sources of carbohydrates are of three types:

a)   **Simple carbohydrates** (Glucose, Fructose, Sucrose): Fruits, Milk, Milk products

b)   **Complex carbohydrates:** Grains Bread, pasta, rice, cereals

c)   **Refined carbohydrates:** Sweeteners, processed foods

Functions

- ➢ Provide energy
- ➢ Improved digestion: Fibre-rich carbohydrates can help prevent digestive problems, such as constipation and indigestion
- ➢ Protect heart: eating whole-grain foods, such as fresh fruit, vegetables, whole wheat, oats, bran and quinoa, gives valuable fiber that protects the heart.
- ➢ Control weight High-fiber foods are generally low in calories as well, so getting enough fibre can help lose weight.

Fats: Fats are one of the essential components along with carbohydrates and proteins. The body needs a certain amount of fat to help the absorption of nutrients and vitamins A, D, E, and K, the fat-soluble vitamins. Fat also fills the fat cells and insulates the body to keep it warm.

Types of fats: These are of two types:

a) Saturated fats

b) Unsaturated Fats

a) Saturated Fats: These fats are solid at room temperature. Foods with a lot of saturated fats are animal products, such as butter, cheese, whole milk, ice cream, cream, and fatty meats. Some vegetable oils, such as coconut, and palm also contains saturated fats. A diet rich in saturated fats increases cholesterol in blood vessels (arteries) Cholesterol is a soft, waxy substance that can raise LDL (bad) cholesterol levels. High LDL cholesterol puts the body at risk for heart attack, stroke, and other major health problems.

b) Unsaturated Fats: Eating unsaturated fats instead of saturated fats can help lower your LDL cholesterol. Most vegetable oils that are liquid at room temperature have unsaturated fats. There are two kinds of unsaturated fats:

- Monounsaturated fats: olive and canola oil
- Polyunsaturated fats: safflower, sunflower, corn, and soy oil

Trans fatty acids are harmful fats that are formed when vegetable oil goes through a process called hydrogenation. This leads the fat to harden and become solid at room temperature.

Trans fats are also used for cooking in some restaurants. They can raise LDL cholesterol

Plant Sources of fats: Olive, peanut, and canola oils, avocados, nuts such as almonds, and hazelnuts. Seeds such as pumpkin and sesame seeds are also rich sources of fat.

Functions of fats:

➢ Source of energy

➢ Vitamin absorption

➢ Insulation of body

Table 3.4 Important facts related with balanced diet

Energy Production	Carbohydrates – 4 calories/gram Proteins- 4 calories/gram Fats- 9 calories/gram
Metabolic Products	Carbohydrates- Glucose Proteins- Amino acids Fats- fatty acids
Excess glucose storage	It is stored as glycogen in liver
Casein	Caesin 80 %, Whey Protein 20%
Essential fatty acids (Only through diet)	Linoleic acid, Linolenic acid

Nutritional Deficiencies

A nutritious and well-balanced diet is critical for overall health. Different nutrients are essential for the body to function properly. A lack or excess of any of the required nutrients in the diet is classified as a nutritional deficit or malnutrition. It is of four different forms:

➢ **Under nutrition** is a condition that occurs when a person eats inadequate food for an extended length of time. It is referred to as starvation in severe circumstances.

➢ **Overeating:** A condition in which a person consumes an excessive amount of food over a lengthy period of time.

➢ **Imbalance:** Disproportion between vital nutrients, with or without extreme nutritional deprivation.

➢ **Specific deficiency** is caused by a relative or absolute absence of a certain nutrient.

Signs of malnutrition: Stunting (low weight for age), wasting (low weight for height), micronutrient deficiency, and obesity are all signs of malnutrition.

Factors causing malnutrition:

The primary cause of malnutrition is a lack of a specific nutrient in the diet, and the secondary cause is that the body is unable to absorb that nutrient due to a medical condition, such as pernicious anemia (inability of the body to absorb vitamin B12), lactose intolerance (the body cannot digest lactose i.e. milk sugar), pancreatic insufficiency (deficiency of pancreatic enzymes that aid in food digestion.

Apart from these, the following socio-economic variables contribute to the incidence of malnutrition:

➤ Poverty is strongly linked to poor nutrition: Household food insecurity can be caused by unemployment, low pay, or a lack of education.

➤ Limited access to a range of foods

➤ Inadequate awareness of recommended dietary practices.

➤ High prevalence of infectious illnesses;

➤ Food consumption patterns (e.g., greater high fat, salt, and sugar); (HFSS)

Major nutritional deficiencies:

1. Protein deficiency

2. Vitamin deficiency

3. Mineral deficit

1. **Protein deficiency:** Protein energy is defined as a lack of proteins, lipids, and carbohydrates. It is the most common kind of malnutrition among children. It causes the following conditions:

   a. Kwashiorkor:

   Occurrence: In 1 to 5-year-old children with a sufficient calorie intake but a significantly protein-deficient diet.

   Characteristics: Due to the accumulation of fluids in the body, the face becomes moon-shaped and the abdomen swells.

   Symptoms include hair loss, dermatitis, tooth loss, and skin depigmentation.

Dietary guidelines for the management of Kwashiorkor:

• The child should be given skimmed milk mixed with boiling water unless he or she is lactose intolerant.

• Include a variety of vegetables in the diet.

   b. Marasmus: It is a Greek word where "maras means to waste away"

   Occurrence: Marasmus can affect anyone but is most common in children. Marasmus can develop if you are severely deficient in nutrients such as calories, proteins, carbohydrates, vitamins, and minerals. It is more prevalent in developing countries.

   Symptoms: Severe muscle atrophy and fat loss throughout the body. This results in significant weight reduction (>85%), dehydration, total muscle loss, anemia, dry skin and brittle hair, and diarrhoea.

Dietary guidelines for the management of Marasmus:

➤ A high-carbohydrate, high-sugar diet that is also high in proteins and important vitamins.

> A lactase-rich diet (lactase is an enzyme) must be provided to youngsters who have developed lactose intolerance.

> To maintain a healthy weight, milk is substituted with vitamin and mineral-rich grains.

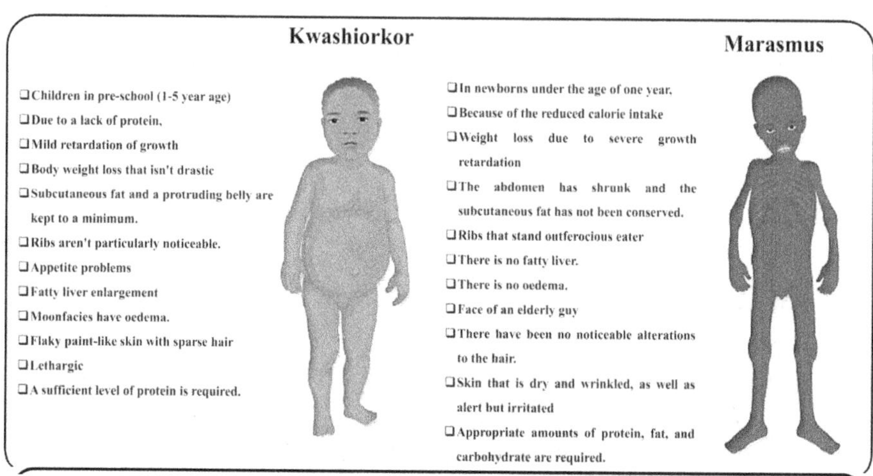

Figure 3.3 Differences between Kwashiorkor and Marasmus

2. **Vitamin deficiencies:** Vitamins are critical for the growth and development of the human body. Despite the fact that they are not required in substantial quantities, their imbalance (absence or excess) causes deficient illnesses.

   a. **Vitamin A deficiency syndrome**: Nyctalopia, or night blindness,

   Symptoms: During the day, people have normal eyesight, but their vision is impaired in the dark.

   Causes: This is caused by a decrease in the pigment rhodopsin, which is found in the retina of the eye and is particularly sensitive to light, and plays an important role in eyesight maintenance.

   Dietary measures: Vitamin A contains the pigment rhodopsin, which may be obtained through foods such as carrots, spinach, lettuce, turnip, papaya, apricot, guava, oil, fish, egg, liver, and milk.

   Vitamin A deficiency can also lead to the development of other disorders.

   > **Xeropthalmia:** The tear duct dries out.

   > **Keratomalacia** is a condition in which the cornea (the transparent area of the eye) softens.

   b. **Vitamin B complex Deficiency**

Table 3.5 Vitamin B-related deficiency disorders.

Vitamin	Name	Function	Deficiency diseases	Symptoms	Dietary Source
Vitamin B1	Thiamine	Essential for the nervous system and required by all the tissues of the body to work properly.	**Beriberi** (body is not able to turn food into fuel)	Disruption of the movement of muscles, numbness of the extremities	Cereals, wheat. carrot. milk
Vitamin B2	Riboflavin	helps in Red blood cells production	**Cheilosis** (cracks in the lips), **glossitis** (inflammation of the tongue), High sensitivity to sunlight	Painful cracks on the corner of the mouth	yogurt milk eggs
Vitamin B3	Niacin	Coenzymes in carbohydrate and protein metabolism (convert nutrients into energy)	**Pellagra**	Dark red rashes resembling sunburn	A balanced diet and Niacin supplement
Vitamin B5	Pantothenic acid	Necessary to make blood cells	**Acne**	Small flesh colored bumps with dark centre on the face	Mushroom Eggs Avacado Whole grains
Vitamin B6	Pyridoxine	Amino acid metabolism	**Seborrheic dermatitis** (eczema), itchy skin, cracks around the mouth	Dry, sensitive Inflamed discolored skin	Potatoes, Starchy food Whole grains Milk
Vitamin B7	Biotin	Does not cause any deficiency in adults	**Impaired growth** in infants	Poor coordination of body movements	

Table 3.5 *Contd....*

Vitamin	Name	Function	Deficiency diseases	Symptoms	Dietary Source
Vitamin B9	Folic acid	It helps to make DNA, repair DNA and produce RBC	**Macrocytic Anaemia** (insufficient concentration of haemoglobin in in the blood) Deficiency during pregnancy can cause **birth defects** in children	Fatigue Palpitation	Fresh fruits (except citrus), vegetables and fortified cereals
Vitamin B12	Cyanocobala min		Neurological damage, **Megaloblastic anaemia** bone marrow produces abnormal-shaped RBC)		Fish, liver, eggs,milk, and curd

c. Vitamin C (ascorbic acid) deficiency:

Vitamin C aids the synthesis of collagen, a protein that aids in the creation of connective tissue. The deficiency of vitamin c causes scurvy (bleeding gums, tooth loss, anemia).

Food sources: Fruits of the citrus family (lemon, orange), apples, grapes

3. Minerals deficiencies:

Minerals are metals, non-metals, and salts extracted from the earth's crust. Minerals do not supply energy but are needed in smaller quantities for physical development and growth; Minerals can be utilized by the human body in complex forms rather than as pure elements. Humans get the majority of their minerals from plants. Major mineral deficiencies are:

a. Iodine deficiency: It is due to the lack of trace element iodine, which is required for the synthesis of the chemical thyroxine, a thyroid hormone. The hormone regulates the body's metabolism.

Deficiency diseases: Hypothyroidism (low thyroid hormone levels) causes inappropriate thyroid gland hypertrophy (Goitre). It can cause developmental delays and mental problems in children.

Food sources of iodine: Seafood, iodized common salt, and dairy products

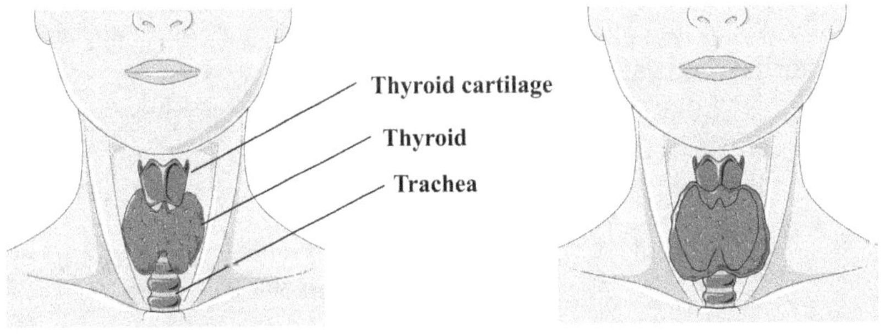

Figure 3.4 Showing Iodine deficiency disorders

b. Calcium: Calcium is required for correct cardiac muscle function, hardening of the bones and teeth, blood coagulation, and muscular contraction.

Deficiency diseases: Osteoporosis (Bones become weak and brittle)

Food sources: Milk, cheese, ragi, sesame

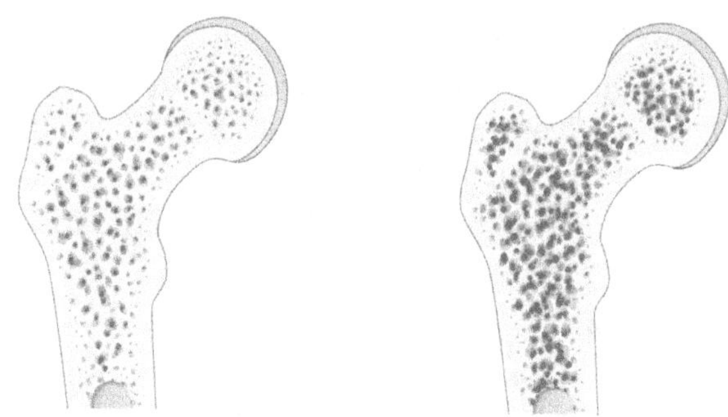

Figure 3.5 Healthy bone and Osteoporosis

c. Iron deficiency: A deficiency in iron is necessary for the development of red blood cells. Deficiency causes anemia (a condition in which hemoglobin concentration is below normal).

Food sources: Milk, eggs, cheese, green vegetables, bajra, apple, banana, egg yolk, fish, and meat.

Malnutrition control strategies

➢ Nutritional Awareness: Educate people on excellent nutrition practices, which include anything from a varied diet to deworming, breastfeeding, cleanliness, and sanitation.

➢ Improved public healthcare in areas with a large migrant population.

➢ Assuring food safety

➢ Public distribution system diversification (Including pulses, oils along with cereals in fair price shops)

➢ Extending the use of salt in food fortification. to bread, oil, and dairy

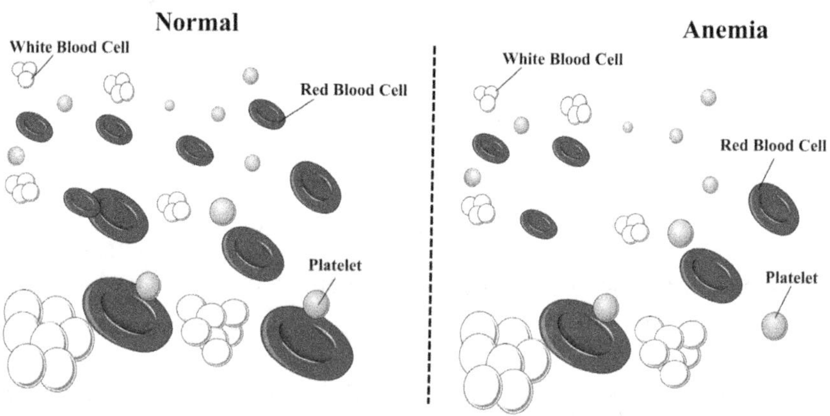

Figure 3.6 Normal cell and anaemic cell

Ill Effects of Junk Food

Junk food and unhealthy diets have become serious threats to health. Food is called junk if it has little or no nutritional value and contains a lot of sugar, fat, or salt (HFSS), and is low in dietary fiber, protein, vitamins, and minerals.

Common examples: Salted snack foods, fried fast food, fizzy drinks, highly processed meals, and high protein foods cooked with saturated fats

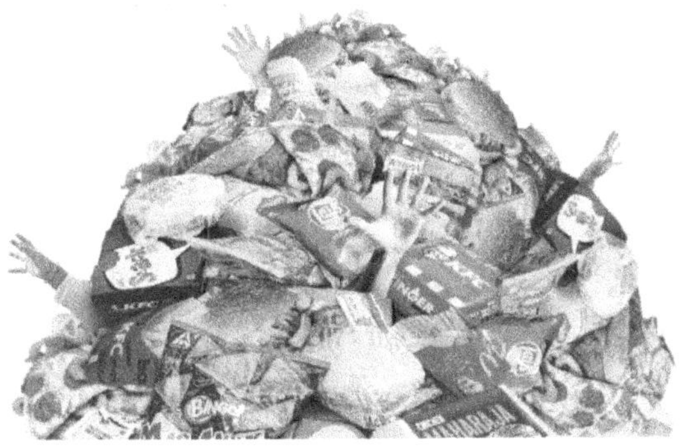

Figure 3.7 Junk food

Ill Effects of Fast/ Junk Food: Consumption of fast food or junk food is harmful to one's health and can contribute to the development and progression of chronic illnesses. A few of them are:

- **Constipation:** Fibre is a major component of our food that helps our digestive tract in flushing wastes from the body. The lack of dietary fiber in the majority of fast foods causes constipation.

- **Heart Problems:** Junk food high in salt and fat may cause inflammation. This inflammation is characterized by the release of cytokines into the circulation which attracts immune cells to the arterial walls, aiding in the formation of plaque, which narrows the arteries. As a result, the risk of heart disease rises.

- **Obesity:** Regular consumption of large quantities of sugar, calories, and fats leads to weight gain and a slowed metabolic rate. This results in obesity, which can lead to health issues such as cardiovascular disease, diabetes, joint pain, and heart disease.

- **Dental issues**: The sugar and carbohydrates in fast food produce acids that can damage tooth enamel and can bring poor dental hygiene. Moreover, the added salt and sugar in fast food sticks to the teeth which may lead to tooth decay and cavities.

- ➢ **Problems with the Skin:** High-carbohydrate, high-sugar fast food contribute to acne and other common skin issues.
- ➢ **Bloating:** The body retains water due to the high salt concentration, which causes the stomach to feel bloated or enlarged.
- ➢ **Anxiety:** A lack of omega-3 fatty acids in junk food can cause stress and unstable mental states. Also, its high carbohydrate content leads to unsteady sugar levels which may lead to, fatigue, depression, and trembling.
- ➢ **Increased cholesterol level:** Mostly junk food is either deep-fried or made from animal products, both of which have a high-fat content. Fat causes an increase in LDL levels and a reduction in HDL (the good cholesterol).
- ➢ **Inadequate child growth and development:** High salt content causes acute inflammation in the hippocampus, in the brain, which is crucial for memory and recognition. Junk meals have a negative impact on children's cognitive development, resulting in a lack of intelligent thinking and chronic degenerative disorders.
- ➢ **Depression:** The gastrointestinal system contains hundreds of billions of bacteria, which connect with the brain via the gut-brain axis. Gut microorganisms generate neurotransmitters such as serotonin and dopamine, which regulate our moods and emotions. Junk food promotes the growth of dangerous bacteria and hinders the release of these neurotransmitters, causing mental health issues like depression.

Regulations: The food safety and standards authority of India FSSAI has released draft regulations for ensuring healthy food for children titled **Food Safety and Standards regulations 2019 (Safe food and healthy diets for school children).** Important regulations are:

- ➢ Advertising and sales ban: It restricts the sale and advertisement of high-fat, high-sugar, and high-salt foods to students within 50 meters of the school.
- ➢ Encourage and promote a healthy, balanced diet: Schools must encourage and promote a healthy, balanced diet at the same time.
- ➢ Food corporations are not allowed to use their logos, brand names, or product names on books or other instructional materials, or on school property such as buildings, buses, or athletic fields.

Calorific and Nutritional Value of Various Foods

Energy is the ability to do work. It is required not only when a person is physically active, but also when the body is resting. Various components of energy expenditure are:

- ➤ **Basal metabolism**: It is the number of calories burnt by the body while at rest. It is determined by the person's muscle (lean) tissue and weight. The more muscle a person has, the faster their metabolism and the more energy their bodies require. Every day, **50 to 80 percent** of the energy used goes to basic metabolic processes (basal metabolism), which allow us to stay warm, breathe, pump blood, and perform a range of other activities

- ➤ **Digestion**: Digestion and subsequent processing of food by the body uses energy and produces heat. This phenomenon known as the thermic effect of food accounts for about **10 percent** of daily energy expenditure.

- ➤ **Physical Activity**: Finally, physical activity, which includes exercise, is the most variable component of energy expenditure, accounting for **20 to 40%** of total energy.

Calorific value: The calorific value of food refers to the number of calories of energy provided by food. The energy is provided and utilized in the following ways:

- ➤ The carbohydrates, fats, and protein (energy-containing macronutrients) are broken down during digestion, releasing energy and nutrients. This energy is expressed in calories (cal) or Kilocalories (kcal).

- ➤ The chemical energy provided by food is ultimately transformed into mechanical energy i.e. the capacity to do work (e.g., muscle contraction). As the intensity of work increases, energy requirements also increase.

- ➤ Some of the energy from these foods is immediately utilized by the body for various physiological processes, while the remaining is stored as fat (adipose tissue) in the body. This varies by age, gender, the intensity of activity, and metabolic rate.

- ➤ To maintain a healthy life, the energy intake (calories) through food should be in balance with energy expenditure.

Nutritional Value:

- ➤ Nutritional value is a measurement of a well-balanced ratio of the fundamental nutrients such as carbohydrates, proteins, fats, vitamins, and minerals in the diet and helps to evaluate the nutritional quality of food, plan a good diet, and live a healthy life.

- ➤ This concept of caloric intake and nutritional value signifies the quality of our diet. According to the ICMR, the average Indian male requires 2200 calories per day, whereas the average Indian female requires 2000 calories per day.

- ➤ The following Table shows the calorie and nutritional content of the most widely eaten Indian foods.

Table 3.6 Calorie and nutritional content of the most widely eaten Indian foods

Food item	Calorific value	Nutritive value		
	calories	Carbohydrates(g)	Proteins(g)	Fats(g)
Milk (300ml)	150	12	8	8
Egg (1)	150	1.1	13	11
Butter biscuit (1)	170	26	3	6
Sweet Tea	100	24	0	0
Rice Bowl	113	31	3	0
Roti (1)	130	90	5	4
Bread (1 piece)	34	6	2	0
Kulcha	291	59	9	2
AlooParantha (1)	154	23	3	9
Masoor Dal (1 bowl)	116	20	9	0
Chana dal (1 bowl)	222	25	8	10
Black grams (1 bowl)	160	14	6	9
Tandoori chicken (100g)	260	13	30	5
PalakPaneer(300g)	320	43	15	0
Samosa (1)	91	24	0	17
Jalebi (1 piece)	150	29	0	3.5
Carrot (large) (1)	30	7	1	0
Potato (100g, boiled)	77	17	1.8	0.1
Almonds (25g) handful	161	2.5	6	14
Peanuts	159	4.52	7.2	14
Apple	47	9.8	0.4	0.4
Banana	89	27	1	0

Fortification of Food

Hidden hunger, or micronutrient deficiencies, contributes to the global disease burden (73%). Over 2 billion people around the globe and the majority in India are micronutrient deficient, including vitamin A, vitamin B_{12}, vitamin D, iron, iodine, folate/folic acid, and zinc. The body doesn't produce micronutrients, so we must consume them through diet. As per the survey conducted by **National Nutrition Monitoring Bureau** (NNMB), the following are the major observations:

➢ The majority of the Indian diet consists of cereal and pulses, with fewer fruits and vegetables.

➢ Micronutrients, particularly iron, calcium, vitamin A, riboflavin, and folic acid, are significantly lacking in Indian diets.

➤ 30 to 90 percent of people of all ages including infants, kids, teenagers, pregnant women, and breastfeeding women are vitamin D deficient.

➤ More than 70% of young children in preschool consume less than 50% of the daily recommended intake (RDA) for iron, vitamin A, and riboflavin.

Deficiencies in essential micronutrients can have a serious effect on health, learning, and productivity. This low productivity results in net economic losses for households, communities, and nations. The prevalence of micronutrient deficiency in India is very high because of 3 main reasons:

➤ Poverty

➤ Lack of access to a variety of food

➤ Lack of knowledge about a variety of dietary intakes and their importance

Prevalence of hidden hunger in India

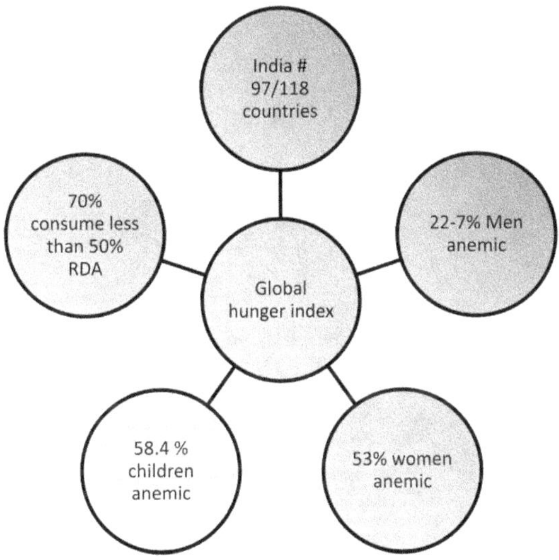

Figure 3.8 The prevalence of hidden hunger in India

Food fortification is one of the most effective health strategies for reducing micronutrient deficiencies and improving general health and well-being.

Food Fortification is defined as the process of intentionally increasing the content of essential micronutrients in food irrespective of whether the nutrients are present originally before processing or to improve the nutritional value of the food.

Types of Food Fortification

➤ **Mass fortification**: Food fortification is done for foods that are widely consumed by the general population e.g. cereals, condiments, milk, oil, and vegetables. It is regulated by the government.

➤ **Targeted fortification**: Foods designed for specific populations such as foods for infants and young children, special food for school children, rations for displaced populations, and special biscuits for pregnant or lactating women.

➤ **Market-driven fortification**: A business-oriented initiative to add/fortify food with certain micronutrients following government rules.

Commonly Fortified foods

One of the fastest and cheapest ways to reach millions of people is through the fortification of staple food and making it available through PDS (Public distribution scheme), ICDS (integrated child development services), and MDM (Mid-day Meals) schemes. The most common are rice, wheat, oil, and milk. Processed and packaged foods are also fortified e.g. Cereals for breakfast, bread, eggs, fruit juice, soy milk, yogurt, and other milk substitutes.

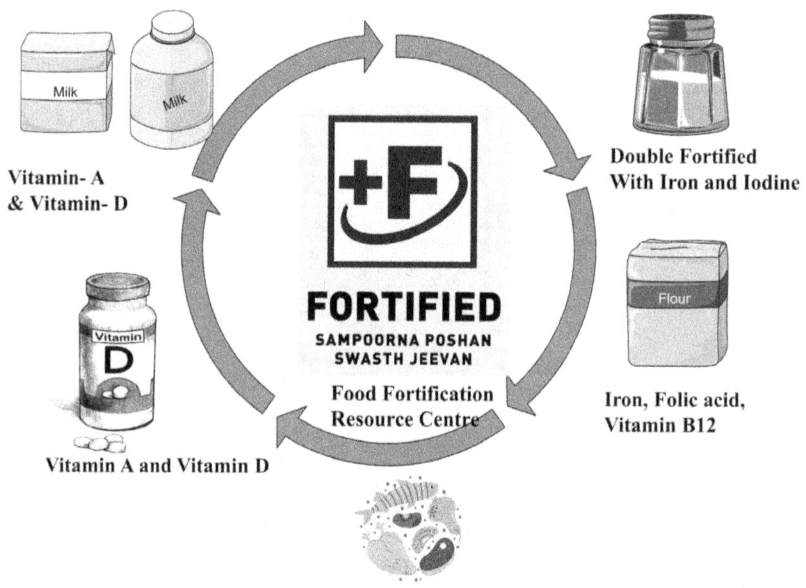

Figure 3.9 Food fortification of widely consumed food

Advantages of fortification

➤ It is a safe and cost-effective approach for improving people's nutrition.

➤ It is a socially and culturally acceptable method of delivering nutrients and does not require dietary or behavioral modifications.

➤ It has no effect on food characteristics including flavor, aroma, or texture.

Fortification regulations: The idea of fortified food is not a new concept in India e.g. Vitamin D in oil & Fats 1953 (vanaspati), Vitamin A in milk, sugar, and wheat Flour, and Iodine in salt (1983/1997). The fortification of food was notified in 2016. The key notifications are:

➢ FSSAI, in October 2016, issued regulations for the **fortification of staple food items** like wheat flour and rice (fortified with Iron, Vitamin B12, and Folic Acid), milk and edible Oil (fortified with Vitamins A and D), and salt (double fortified with Iodine and Iron) to reduce the high burden of micronutrient malnutrition

➢ In 2017, India's **National Nutritional strategy, 2017,** listed food fortification as one of the interventions to address anemia and iodine deficiencies.

➢ In 2018, the Food Safety and Standards Authority of India (FSSAI) issued new laws that made food fortification mandatory for all brands in the nation and created a new **+F mark for fortified foods**

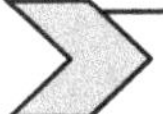

3.4   Food Safety

➢ Food is the main determinant of a population's health, nutritional status, and productivity. Access to nutritious and safe food is critical to public health. It is essential that the food we consume is healthy and safe.

➢ Food safety, nutrition, and food security are closely linked. Unsafe food may lead to disease and malnutrition particularly affecting infants, young children, the elderly, pregnant women, and the sick.

➢ Unsafe food containing harmful bacteria, viruses, parasites, or chemical substances, causes more than 200 diseases ranging from diarrhea to cancers.

➢ A large proportion of foodborne disease incidents are caused by foods improperly prepared or mishandled at home, in food service establishments, or at markets.

➢ Diarrheal diseases are the most common illnesses resulting from the consumption of contaminated food, causing 550 million people to fall ill and 230000 deaths every year.

➢ Food-borne infections cause not only diseases but also can damage trade and tourism, income loss, unemployment, increase litigation, and limit economic progress. The safety of food promotes national economies

FSSAI (Food Safety and Standard Act 2006) defines food safety as the **'assurance that food is acceptable for human consumption according to its intended use'**

Major contaminants of food: Three major hazards that may contaminate food and lead to a breach of food safety are:

1. **Physical Hazard:** Presence of dirt, dust, metal, hair, etc. that contaminate food

2. **Chemical Hazard:** Presence of pesticides, heavy metals, allergens, etc
3. **Biological Hazard:** Presence of microorganisms (mainly), parasites.

Chemical Contamination

Table 3.7 Health effects of Chemical contaminants

Type of chemical contaminant	Examples	Health effects
Naturally occurring toxins	Poisonous mushrooms, molds, growing on grains.	Long-term exposure can affect the immune system and normal development, or cause cancer.
Organic pollutants: These are unwanted by-products of industrial processes and waste incineration.	Dioxins and polychlorinated biphenyls (PCBs)	Long-term exposure can affect the immune system and normal development, or cause cancer.
Heavy metals: Contamination in food occurs mainly through pollution of air, water, and soil.	Lead, cadmium, and mercury)	

Microbial Contamination

Table 3.8 Health effects of Microbial Contaminants

Microorganism	Causative organism	Health effects
Bacteria	*Salmonella:* eggs, poultry, and other products of animal origin	Nausea, vomiting, abdominal pain, and diarrhea
	Campylobacter raw milk, raw or undercooked poultry, and drinking water	Nausea, vomiting, abdominal pain, and diarrhea
	Escherichia coli, Unpasteurized milk, undercooked meat, and fresh fruits and vegetables	Fever, headache, nausea, vomiting, abdominal pain and
	Listeria, unpasteurized dairy products and various ready-to-eat foods	Miscarriage in pregnant women or death of newborn babies.
	Vibrio cholerae contaminated water or food	abdominal pain, vomiting, and profuse watery diarrhea, which may lead to severe dehydration and possibly death
Virus	Hepatitis A	vomiting, watery diarrhea and abdominal pain, Jaundice
Parasites	Tapeworms,	Taeniasis
	Entamoeba histolytica	Amoebiasis
	Giardia	Giardiasis

The first two risks (physical and chemical) may be removed during the screening and processing of raw materials, but it is challenging to control microbes because food provides nutritional support for the organisms and promotes their growth. As a result, in addition to factors like self-degradation through chemical reactions, the majority of food spoilages are also related to microbiological spoilages.

Policies to address Food safety: The following policies may be beneficial

➢ There should be adequate **food systems and infrastructures** (e.g. laboratories) to manage food safety risks along the entire food chain.

➢ Food safety should be integrated into wider food policies and programs (e.g., nutrition and food security).

WHO Five keys to safer food created in 2001 help countries build capacity to prevent, detect and manage food-borne risks. These *five keys to safer food* are particularly useful in the prevention of food-borne diseases and provide the basis for educational initiatives that train food workers and educate consumers. They are simple and practical, and they must be used by people at homes and in restaurants.

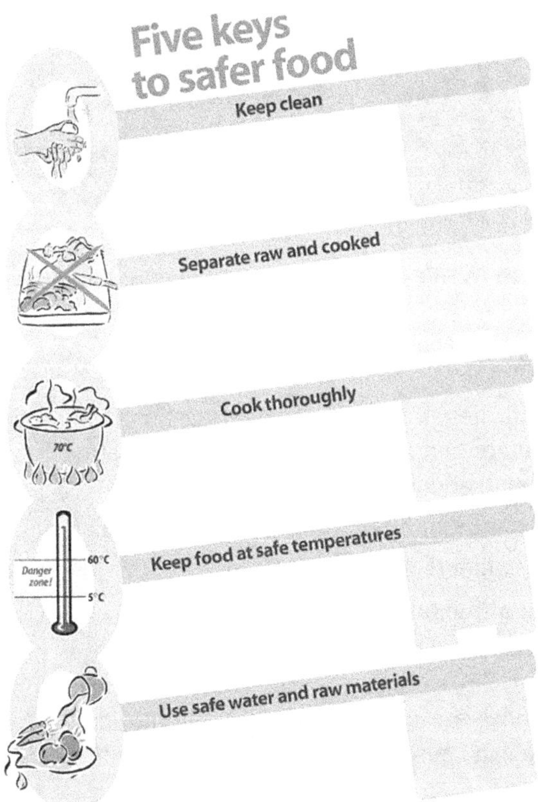

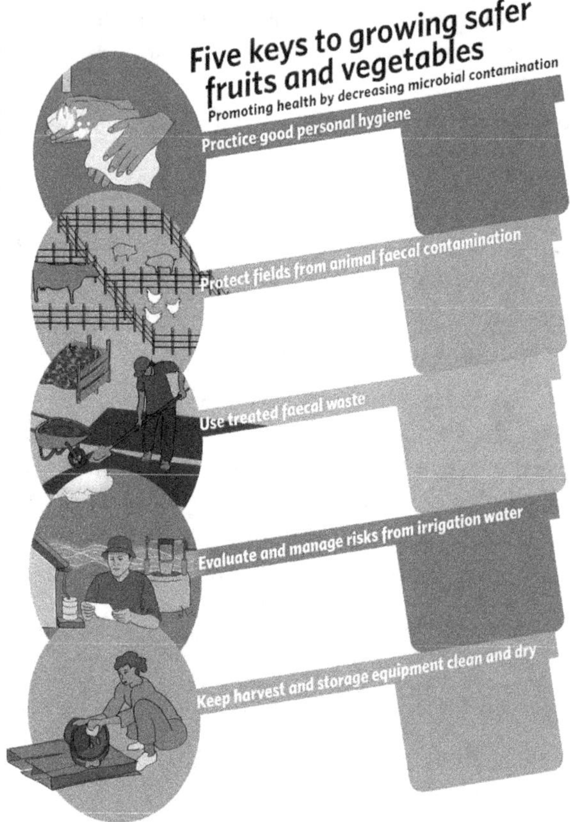

Figure 3.10 WHO's five keys for safer food and for growing safer fruits and vegetables

Food Adulteration

Adulteration is an illegal process of lowering the quality of any product by adding inferior ingredients. The practice of adulterating food is called food adulteration. It can be done in the following ways:

➢ Addition, substitution, mixing of inferior quality material.

➢ Extraction of valuable ingredients.

➢ False labeling of the product (concealing quality).

➢ Biological and chemical contamination during the period of growth, storage, processing, transport, and distribution of food products. The added substances are called adulterants. Food adulteration deceives the consumer and can cause serious risks to their health.

Types of food contaminants: Food is adulterated at every stage, from preparation to consumption. The major contaminants of food are:

➢ Physical contaminants
➢ Biological contaminants
➢ Chemical contaminants

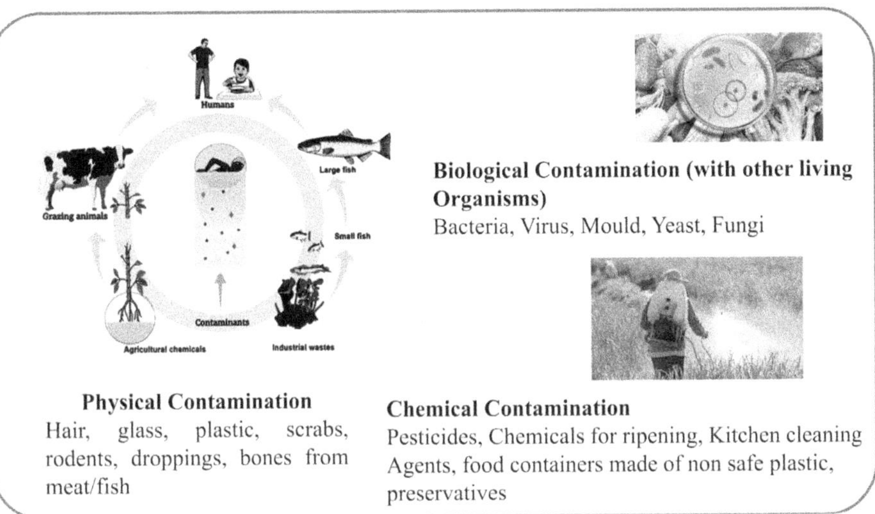

Figure 3.11 Different types of contaminants

Causes of food adulteration: The main reasons for food adulteration are:

➢ The profit motive of traders.
➢ To increase the quantity of food production and sales.
➢ Illiteracy of the general public for proper food consumption.
➢ Lack of effective food laws.

Types of food adulteration

1. **Intentional adulteration:** The adulterants are intentionally inserted to increase profit (Sand, marble fragments, stones, chalk powder, and other similar materials).

2. Adulterants are detected in food as a result of neglect, ignorance, or a lack of suitable facilities. (Packaging concerns include insect larvae, droppings, pesticide residues, etc.).

3. **Metallic impurities adulteration:** When metallic substances are purposely or unintentionally introduced to a beverage. (Arsenic, pesticides, lead from drinking water, etc).

4. **Packaging Hazard-** The materials used to package the food may interact with and mix with the food's ingredients, resulting in packaging risks.

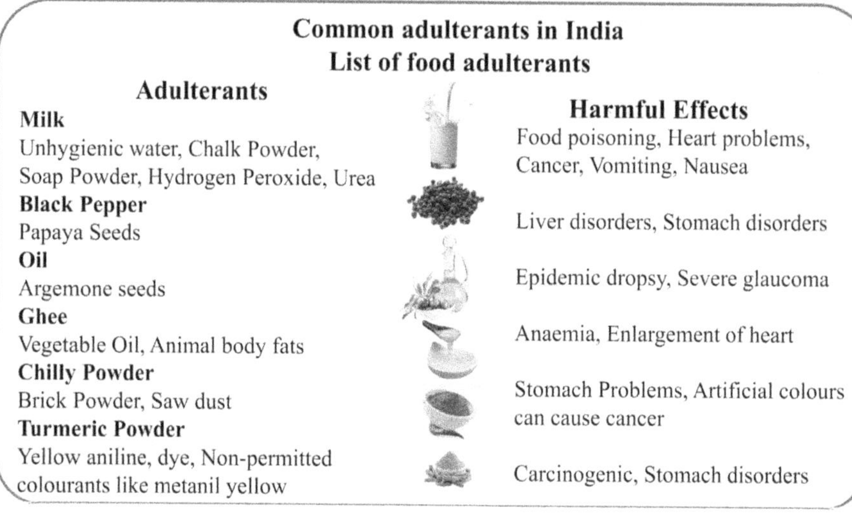

Figure 3.12 Common adulterants in India

Standards to protect against food Adulteration: The Indian government has established various guidelines to ensure the quality of food goods. FSSAI (Food Safety and Standard Authority of India) is a government license number that stands for food safety and performs food testing for various adulterants in Indian markets. Different quality marks are approved by the government to ensure the quality and purity of food products e.g. Agmark, ISI, FPO, Organic farm food.

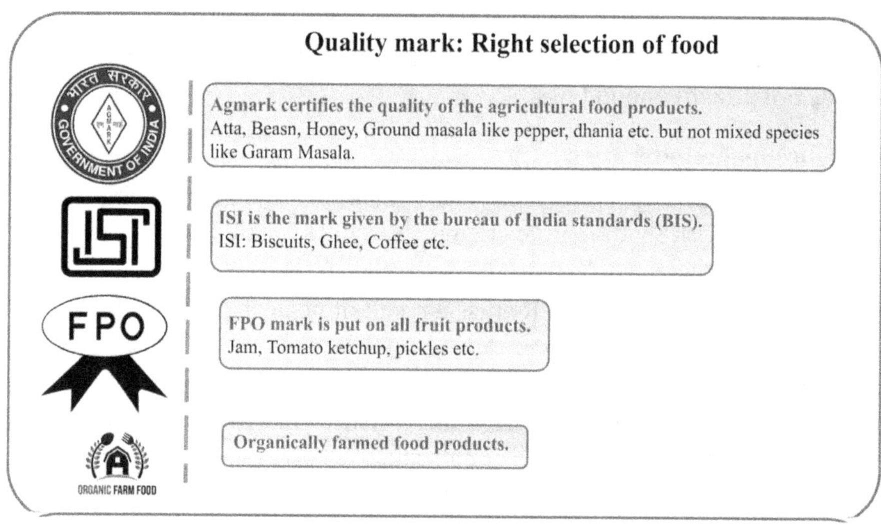

Figure 3.13 Quality Marks-Right selection of food

Artificial Ripening

India ranks second in fruit production in the world after China. Mangoes, grapes, walnuts, pomegranates, bananas are largely exported. Ripening of fruit is a natural, physiological process by which fruits attain their desirable flavor, quality, color, texture and taste.

Artificial ripening: It is the process by which ripening of fruits is controlled and the product may be achieved as per requirement by controlling the different parameters.

Generally, 80% fruits are ripened artificially through ripening agents. A faster and uniform ripening with increased organoleptic qualities is achieved but, nutritive value and shelf life of such items are depreciated. Additionally, various health risks are associated with the use of artificial ripeners.

Based on ripening process there are two types of fruits:

> *Non - Climacteric fruit:* Fruits once harvested do not ripen further. So, such fruits are harvested once they are fully ripened. For example Orange, grapes, watermelon, strawberry, litchi blackberry etc.

> **Climacteric fruits** continue to ripen after harvest e.g. Mango, banana, apple, kiwi, plums, pears, guava etc. So such fruits are harvested hard and green. They emit a sufficient amount of **ethylene** (naturally released plant growth regulator) that favors ripening along with increased respiration rate.

Ethylene (C2H4): It is a natural plant growth regulator. It is a gaseous hormone naturally produced in fruit. It acts as stimulating or regulating enzyme for the ripening of fruit. As fruits ripe they release more and more ethylene that fastens ripening process. These fruits cannot withstand rigorous transport and handling. The only safe and worldwide accepted method is using ethylene. Commercially, it is very expensive, so traders use other chemicals.

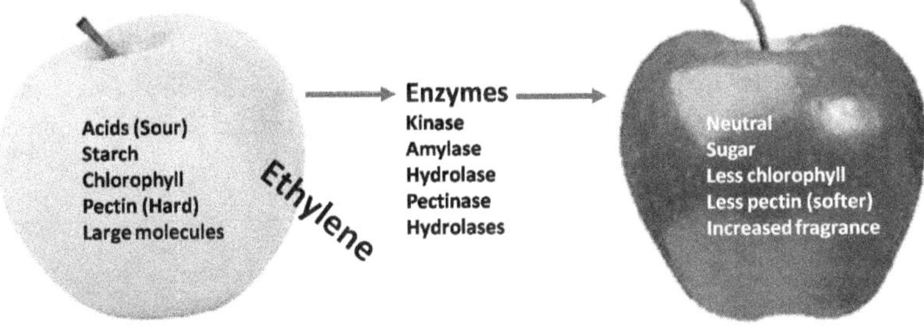

Figure 3.14 Ethylene ripening

Considering the hazardous effects, the use of ripeners like calcium carbide, and ethephon must be strictly monitored and controlled. It is not solely the responsibility of the Government. People must also become aware and avoid consuming contaminated fruits.

Table 3.9 Health effects of artificial ripening agents

S.No	Ripening agent	Mechanism	Health effects
1.	**Carbide** Harmful and banned in India	A pouch of powder is kept in fruit containers. It reacts with moisture to produce acetylene gas (Carbide gas) that acts as a ripening agent.	Carbide contains traces of Arsenic and Phosphorous hydride which are carcinogenic. Symptoms: diarrhea difficulty in swallowing, burning sensation of chest and abdomen, burning in the eyes and skin, permanent eye damage, ulcers on skin, weakness, thirst, irritation, . respiratory problems, sore throat, cough and shortness of breath.
2.	**Ethephon** Less harmful, safe, and approved in India	Acts by producing ethylene. Commercially available as **Floral, Cepa.** Fruits are dipped in its solutions and kept in airtight containers until ripe.	Associated with cholinergic side effects, anemia, and some respiratory problems
3.	**Ethylene glycol**	Ethylene reacts with hydrogen peroxide to produce the agent ethylene glycol, which when diluted with water can hastens fasting, particularly in a cold climate	Ethylene glycol if ingested is poisonous and may cause kidney failure.

Use of Pesticides

The industrialization of agriculture, with a focus on higher productivity, profits, and disease prevention, has increased the chemical burden on natural ecosystems. Pesticides are chemical substances or mixtures of chemicals that are mostly employed in agriculture or public health programs to protect plants from pests, weeds, or diseases, and humans from vector-borne diseases such as malaria, dengue fever, etc.

Types of Pesticides: There are various types of pesticides e.g.

- ➢ **Insecticides:** These pesticides reduce the destruction and contamination of growing and harvested crops by insects and their eggs.

- ➢ **Herbicides:** Also known as weed killers, herbicides improve crop yields.

- ➢ **Rodenticides:** These are important for controlling the destruction and contamination of crops by rodent-borne diseases.

- ➢ **Fungicides.** This type of pesticide is especially important for protecting harvested crops and seeds from fungal rot.

Pesticides use in India: The green revolution introduced chemical fertilizers and chemical pesticides.

Table 3.10 List of most common chemical pesticides

Chemical Pesticides	
Organophosphate Pesticides	Parathion, malathion, and methyl parathion
Carbamate Pesticides	Bendiocarb, carbaryl, methomyl, and propoxur
Organochlorine Insecticides	DDT and chlordane.
Pyrethroid Pesticides	Pyrethrin, permethrin, resmethrin, and sumithrin

Benefits of Pesticides: Pesticide use increases and stabilizes crop productivity, protects the nutritional integrity of foodstuffs, promotes storage to ensure year-round supplies, and produces appealing food products.

Major Problem: Unfortunately, there is significant misuse, abuse, and overuse of pesticides, which causes a serious issue in form of pesticide residue in food, the environment, and biological systems.

Pesticide residues: When a crop is treated with a pesticide, a very small amount of the pesticide, or its 'metabolites' or 'degradation products', can remain in the crop even after it is harvested. This is known as the '**residue**'.

Pesticide residues can be found in fresh or canned fruits and vegetables, or in processed food and drink derived from the treated crop. Animal products like milk and meat may also contain pesticide residues.

The pesticide residues can arise from:
- ➢ Use/overuse of a legally permitted pesticide on a crop that is close to harvest.
- ➢ Illegal use of a pesticide that is not approved for that crop.

➤ Incorrect treatment of insecticides after harvest to prevent pest infestation during storage or transport.

➤ Residues can sometimes be found in the environment or from other 'indirect' sources. These residues ultimately pollute water, air, soil, food, and the ecosystem and have a profound effect on public health and increase the burden of disease.

Health effects of pesticide residues are:

1. **Acute health effects**: Itching, burning, headache, nausea, fatigue, vomiting.

2. **Reproductive impact**: early puberty, disturbed menstrual cycle, decrease sperm count, or impaired fertility in males

3. **Hormone disruption**: mimic naturally produced hormones and disrupt hormonal functions and metabolism disorders.

4. **Birth Defects:** birth defects like limb reduction defects, and increased risk of cleft palate in children born to pesticide applicators.

5. **Neurological effects:** The risk of developing Parkinson's disease and dementia, reduced IQ and learning disability, poorer memory, and less skill in drawing figures. less stamina, Neurotoxicity due to inhibition of cholinesterase enzyme, lack of neuromuscular coordination, poorer eye-hand coordination,

6. **Cancer:** leukemia, lymphoma, brain, kidney, breast, prostate, pancreas, liver, lung, and skin cancers, leukemia, neuroblastoma, Wilms tumor, soft-tissue sarcoma, Ewing's sarcoma, Non-Hodgkins's lymphoma, and cancers of the brain, colorectum, and testes.

7. **Immunotoxicity:** Impaired immune system, autoimmune disorders, and allergic reactions.

Pesticide residue in food can be avoided by:

➤ Promoting search for biopesticides.

➤ Educating farmers about alternative pest control methods.

➤ Introducing better pesticide application technology.

➤ Promotion of alternative farming methods, including organic farming and hydroponics for the production of grains and vegetables.

➤ Organic foods are likely to have lower levels of residues than non-organic foods.

Genetically Modified Organism

Genetically refers to **genes, Modified** implies that some **change** has been made and the last word is **Organism** (an 'organism' isn't just a plant; it refers to all living things, including bacteria and fungi).

Genetic engineering

Researchers isolate a gene from an organism that has the trait they want to impart to a plant.

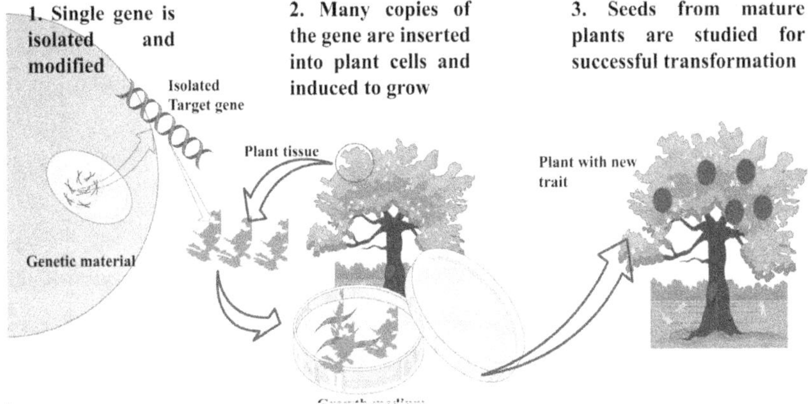

Figure 3.15 The process of genetic modification of plants

Traditional breeding in fields involves mixing all of the genes from two different sources while the genetic modification is targeted and takes place in laboratories. This process of combining inter-species genes is called recombinant DNA technology. The desirable genes are inserted in a single cell to create a new genetically-altered cell with enhanced nutritional, productive, and ecological value. Once this single cell has been modified, it is treated with naturally occurring plant hormones to stimulate growth and development until it becomes a whole plant. Because this new plant was derived from a single cell with the inserted gene, all of the cells in the regenerated plant contain that new gene.

Advantages of Genetically Modified foods: GM foods have the following properties:

➢ More productive.

➢ Comparatively more nutritional value and flavour.

➢ The genetically modification of food eliminates allergy causing properties in some foods.

➢ Pest, weed, and disease resistance.

➢ GM crops are capable to thrive in areas with poor soil or adverse weather conditions.

➢ They are more environmentally friendly because they require fewer herbicides and pesticides.

➢ GM foods are more resistant and stay ripe for longer periods of time, allowing them to be shipped over long distances or kept on store shelves for longer periods of time.

➢ GM crops are an answer to feeding the world's growing population because they can be grown on comparatively small areas of land.

Disadvantages of Genetically Modified foods

➢ GM foods are sold without evaluating their health risks sufficiently.

➢ Many GM companies **do not label their foods as being GM foods**. Not labeling is wrong and unfair to the consumers who should have the right to know what they are buying.

➢ Some people might have moral or religious objections to buying such foods.

➢ Herbicide-resistant and pesticide-resistant crops could give rise to super-weeds and super-pests that would need newer, stronger chemicals to destroy them.

➢ GM crops could cross-pollinate with nearby non-GM plants and create ecological problems.

➢ GM technology companies patent their crops. The seeds are **expensive and farmers have to buy the seeds from the companies every time.**

➢ The new technology also interferes with their traditional agricultural ways which may be more suited to their conditions.

GM technology can also be used on microorganisms. For example, bacteria can be genetically modified to produce medicines that can cure diseases A commonly used medicine that comes from a genetically modified source is insulin, which is used to treat diabetes, but there are many others.

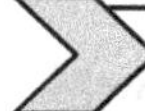

3.5   Supplements

Diet and physical exercise are thought to be crucial in sustaining health and avoiding illness. Cardiovascular disease, some forms of cancer, osteoporosis, diabetes, obesity, high blood pressure, depression, stress, and anxiety are all reduced by regular physical activity. Taking dietary supplements is now thought to offer health-promoting properties.

Dietary Supplements

➢ These are the foods that are consumed in addition to a regular diet to provide additional nutrients. They are used to make up for nutritional deficiencies and support certain biological functions.

➢ They are not medicinal products and as such cannot exert a pharmacological, immunological, or metabolic action. Therefore unlike drugs, their use is not intended to treat or prevent diseases in humans or to modify physiological functions.

➢ In higher concentrations, they may cause drug-like responses. As a result, they should only be used as needed to complement the diet or as directed.

➢ They contain one or more ingredients like vitamins, minerals, amino acids, herbs, and botanicals in form of pills, capsules, tablets, or liquids, powders, and beverages and are labeled as dietary supplements. The most commonly used supplements are vitamins, minerals, omega-3 fish oil, Ginkobiloba extract, and soy protein.

Food items that are fortified with nutrients such as vitamins and minerals to ensure proper nutrient levels are not considered dietary supplements.

Types of Dietary Supplements:

1. Herbs and Botanicals

2. Vitamins

3. Minerals

4. Sports nutrition supplements (e.g. protein powder)

5. Meal replacement

6. Specialty products (Amino acids, hormones, fish oil).

Table 3.11 Categories of nutrients and their sources

Category and class of Nutrients	Type of dietary supplement	Most Common Requirement	Natural Source
Micronutrients	Vitamins	Vitamin D, B_{12}	Sunlight, cheese, egg yolk, fish, meat, fish egg, milk
	Minerals	Calcium, Iron	Nuts, cereals, Meat
Macronutrient	Fatty Acids, Proteins, Amino Acids	Linoelic acid (ALA), Eicosapentaenoic acid (EPA), Docosahexaenoic acid (DHA)	Flaxseed, soybean, and canola oil, sea Fish
Herbs	Botanical	-	Ginkgo biloba, garlic
Phytochemicals	Lycopene Isoflavone	-	Guava, tomatoes watermelon, soy, Beans, Peas
others		Probiotics, Glucosamine, Melatonin, Omega 3 Fatty Acids	Yogurt, pickles, shellfish, cherries, fish

Health benefits of dietary supplements:

➢ Reduce aging e.g. Garlic, ginseng

➢ Reduce the risk of cancer e.g. Glutathione, lycopenes

➢ Maintenance of joint functioning e.g. Vitamin D, Glucosamine

➢ Improve cognitive functions e.g. Brahmi, Ginko biloba

➢ Protect from cardiovascular diseases e.g. Garlic

➢ Improve reproductive health e.g. Ginseng, Ashwagandha

➢ Increase the immunity e.g. Ashwagandha

➢ Maintenance of bone mineral density Calcium, Vitamin D, Omega 3 Fatty acids

Table 3.12 Important dietary supplements, their usage and potential risk

Dietary supplement	Usage	Probable risks
Multivitamin/multimineral , vitamin and minerals	Beneficial in patients of nutritional deficiency.	**Overconsumption of Vit B6:** photosensitivity and neurotoxicity. **Overconsumption of Vit E:** bleeding disorders, diarrhea, weakness, blurred vision and gonadal dysfunction. **Excess vitamin A supplementation:** low bone mineral density and increased fracture risk. If consumed during pregnancy leads to congenital abnormalities.
Fish oil and Omega3 Fatty acids	Keeps lipid levels in control, possess anti-cancer and cardioprotective effects	Promotes bleeding in patients taking anticoagulant medications such as warfarin as fish oil consumption increases Vit A levels.
Protein powders and Infant formulas Contain dairy proteins like casein, whey, and vegetable proteins isolated from soy	Used by athletes, Bodybuilders, or patients with protein deficiency and low body weight. Used as weight loss supplements	**Soy proteins:** produce reproductive toxicity, infertility, and estrogen-responsive cancers such as breast and endometrial cancer. **Milk proteins:** excessive consumption may result in ketosis. Some people are allergic to milk proteins
Botanical Supplements consist of a mixture of organic compounds		**Kava kava**; Produces liver toxicity by increasing oxidative stress and mitochondrial dysfunction. **Valerian:** jaundice **Milk thistle:** Iron overload **Garlic and ginkgo biloba:** excessive bleeding

Regulation of dietary supplements: Dietary supplements have questionable safety profiles as these can be sold in the market without the support of clinical trials. FDA does not assess the quality and its effects on the body. These are regulated by the **Food Safety and Standards Authority of India** (FSSAI) which was established under the Food Safety and Standards Act, 2006. According to this,

'The manufacturers are responsible for the product's purity, and it is mandatory to list ingredients and their amounts accurately on the label. But there's no regulatory agency that makes sure that labels match what's in the bottles.'

Nutraceuticals

Food provides nutrients that help to nourish our bodies and keep our systems in proper working condition. There are certain foods that give additional health benefits to humans, such as disease prevention and treatment. Such health-promoting foods are generally classified into 2 major categories:

1. Nutraceuticals

2. Functional foods

1. **Nutraceuticals** (nutrients + pharmaceuticals):

➢ Nutrients (nourishing food components) and pharmaceuticals (medical drugs) provide health benefits. So nutraceuticals are health-promoting foods.

➢ The term nutraceutical was coined by Stephen L. De Felice in 1989 and defined as any substance that may be regarded as a food or a component of a diet that provides medical or health benefits, including the prevention and treatment of illness.

➢ These products may include isolated nutrients or purified nutrients from food sources / herbal products, as well as processed products such as cereals, soups, and beverages.

➢ In India, nutraceuticals are food components made from herbal or botanical raw materials that are used to prevent or cure many kinds of acute and chronic disease conditions.

➢ Nutraceuticals are no longer merely used in preventive and curative treatment; they are also used to lose weight, improve hair growth, attain glowing skin, and treat diseases such as thyroid, nail disorders, diabetes, arthritis, and others.

Classification: Nutraceuticals are characterized in the following ways:

➢ **Traditional/Natural nutraceuticals:** Herbals, phytochemicals, probiotics, nutraceutical enzymes.

➢ **Non-traditional nutraceuticals**: Fortified fish oil capsules, herb extracts, glucosamine and chondroitin sulfate pills, lutein-containing multivitamin tablets, and antihypertensive pills that contain fish protein-derived peptides.

Natural extracts

1. **Turmeric:** The bioactive components of turmeric, called curcuminoids, are used for their anti-inflammatory and anti-arthritic properties.

2. **Garlic:** Allicin, the primary ingredient in garlic, has been shown to lower blood fat and cholesterol levels, hence lowering the risk of heart disease. The antibacterial and antiviral properties of garlic are also used to treat cold and respiratory infections.

3. **Ginger:** The extract of ginger contains gingerol which has proven to be useful in treating nausea, including motion sickness and morning sickness.

4. **Ginkgo biloba:** The extract of *Ginkgo biloba* contains terpene-lactones and is commonly used to treat poor blood circulation.

5. **Ginseng:** The extract of Ginseng contains ginsenosides which are generally used to treat fatigue.

Nutraceutical industry in India: Dabur, Himalaya, and the Baidyanath group have a long history of producing herbal and ayurvedic medicines in India. Patanjali, a new and more dominating entry, is also playing a critical role in popularizing Ayurveda and boosting the nutraceutical business.

Functional Food

➤ Functional foods are often ingested as part of a regular diet, but in addition to providing nutrients, they can help to lower the risk of chronic illnesses including cancer, hypertension, and renal failure.

➤ Tomatoes have lycopene which is a potent antioxidant that helps to eliminate harmful substances from our systems and prevent damage to the vital organs. Other examples of functional food are: soybeans, salmon, oatmeal, cereal bran (wheat, rice), and tea are all examples of useful foods (green and black).

➤ Besides from daily meals, functional foods are prepared by food processing also e.g. yogurt drinks (pre-and probiotics, fortified drinks), functional milk (extra calcium, omega-3, and vitamin-fortified drinks), juices (vitamins and omega-3 fortified drinks), functional waters (vitamin and mineral fortified drinks, sports and energy drinks, herbal drinks, and health and wellness drinks).

Food Supplements

No single food contains all of the essential nutrients our body needs. Each food provides our body with certain nutrients. Eating/selecting only one type of food or eliminating a food group from the diet, despite eating enough calories, can increase the risk of diet-related negative health conditions. Food supplements are an effective means of getting nutrients if the deficiency is caused by the following:

1. **Lactose intolerance:** It is due to the body's inability to digest lactose, a sugar present in milk and other dairy products. Avoiding milk can result

in a lack of calcium and vitamin D since milk and milk products are the most prevalent sources of calcium.

Supplements: Many non-lactose foods, such as broccoli and leafy green vegetables, oranges, almonds, dry beans, tofu, soy milk, and soft-boned fish are alternative sources of calcium.

2. **Gluten intolerance:** It is the inability of the body to digest or break down gluten. Gluten is a protein found in all wheat, rye, oats, and barley varieties. When individuals with celiac illness consume gluten, the absorptive villi of the small intestine are damaged, blocking the absorption of numerous vital nutrients. The long-term consequences of untreated celiac disease can be fatal. However, with a gluten-free diet, the intestinal lining will recover entirely, allowing the majority of patients to live normal, healthy life. Not following a gluten-free diet may result in thiamine, riboflavin, iron, calcium, folate, vitamin D, and magnesium deficits.

Supplements: Foods like black beans, lentils, leafy greens, mushrooms, fatty fish, and almonds.

3. **Vegetarian/Vegan Diet:** Vegans eat only plant-based foods and avoid animal products (milk, dairy, eggs, and sometimes honey and gelatin). Eliminating animal products increases the risk of protein, minerals (particularly iron, calcium, and zinc), vitamin B12, and vitamin D deficiencies.

Supplements: Plant-based sources of all nutrients, such as walnuts, chia seeds, mushrooms, soy milk, lentils, cashews, and leafy greens can be incorporated into the diet.

4. **Ethnic Food choices:** Staple cereal grains like wheat, maize, barley, and rice are the major grains eaten worldwide and provide the most accessible form of energy. People eating only one type of grain are at the risk of developing develop nutritional diseases e.g.

   ➢ **Maize**: When maize is the main food source then the risk of developing pellagra is high as maize is low in niacin and tryptophan. Furthermore, the niacin in maize cannot be absorbed in the intestine unless the maize is treated with alkali.

   ➢ **Rice:** Rice-eating population develops thiamine deficiency.

   ➢ **Wheat**: Wheat is one of the major grains eaten worldwide but wheat processing remarkably affects the Zn intake of people because aleurone in bran layers of wheat is usually removed during processing.

Supplements: Chickpeas, lentils, beans, hemp seeds, almonds, quinoa, rice, oat, and dairy products (milk, eggs, cheese).

5. Keto diet: It is a low-carb, high-fat, and moderate-protein diet that helps people to lose weight and control blood glucose levels. The body breaks down fats for energy which leads to weight loss. Low carb diet can lead to deficiencies in thiamine, folate, calcium, vitamin E, and magnesium.

Supplements: Flax seeds, peanuts, avocado, broccoli, spinach, green bell paper, red bell paper, cabbage, tofu, soybeans, spinach, and peanuts.

Drug-Food Interactions

A drug-food interaction occurs when the food we eat and the medicine we take interfere with one another. Drugs do not combine in the body to produce chemical reactions instead; food or supplement may affect the stay of medication in the body. A food-drug interaction can show major clinical effects in the following ways:

➤ Decreased availability of a drug in the body, which put the risk of treatment failure,

➤ An increased availability increases the risk of adverse events and may even precipitate toxicities.

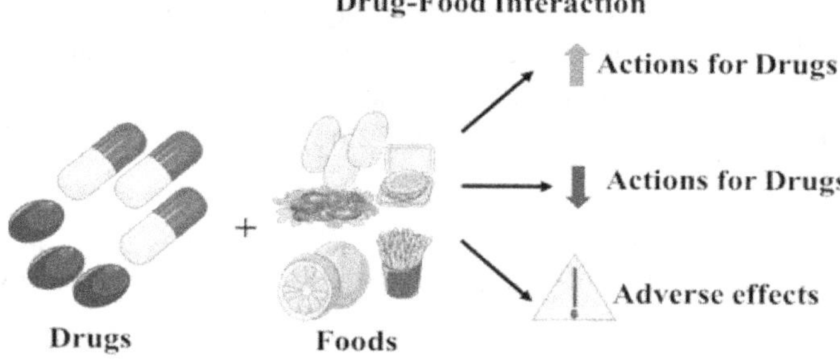

Figure 3.16 Drug- Food Interaction

Types of Drug-nutrient Interactions: drug-nutrient interactions fall into two broad categories

➤ Pharmaceutical interactions

➤ Pharmacological interactions

Pharmaceutical Interactions: This refers to the biochemical or physical interactions between drug formulation and the dietary element. It can occur through different chemical processes e.g. hydrolysis, oxidation, neutralization, precipitation, and complexation. These responses often occur when the interacting agents come into direct physical contact and occur prior to the nutrients or drugs are administered.

Pharmacological Interactions: These kind of drug-food interactions are identified as reactions that occur inside the body. Pharmacological interactions are classified as:

➢ Pharmacodynamic interactions

➢ Pharmacokinetic interactions.

Pharmacodynamic Interactions: The pharmcodynamic interactions may lead to either increase or decrease in the therapeutic effect of the drug. As a result, there may be an increase in toxicity of the drug or failure of therapy.

Pharmacokinetic Interactions: These interactions may have an effect on the bioavailability, efficacy, and elimination of the drug. Many types of food have a significant effect on the action of drugs by affecting the absorption, metabolism, and excretion of the drugs.

The interaction with food may result in an increase or decrease in the effect of the drug by affecting

1. Absorption of drug

2. Distribution of the drug within the body.

3. Metabolism of the drug

4. Elimination of the drug

Effect on drug absorption:

➢ Food acts to limit drug absorption by slowing digestion, binding to minerals contained in food, or binding to food particles.

➢ The absorption of some drugs is increased by food. Therefore, these drugs are taken with food in order to increase their concentration in the body and, ultimately, their effect. Conversely, when a drug's absorption is reduced by food, the drug is taken on an empty stomach.

Effect on drug metabolism and elimination:

➢ The kidney and liver are critical sites of possible drug interactions as most drugs are processed in the liver and removed through the kidneys.

➢ The cytochrome P450 enzymes are a group of enzymes in the liver that are responsible for the metabolism of most drugs. They are, therefore, often involved in drug interactions.

➢ Drugs and certain foods can increase or reduce the activity of these enzymes, influencing the concentration of drugs metabolized by these enzymes. An increase in the activity of these enzymes decreases the concentration and effect of the administered medication. In contrast, a reduction in enzyme activity increases drug concentration and the effect of the drug.

Common Food-Drug Interactions: Food and drinks do not mix with certain prescription drugs or over-the-counter drugs (OTC), herbal products, and even dietary supplements. They can cause delayed, decreased, or enhanced absorption of the drugs. There are 3 categories

➤ Food – Drug interaction
➤ Nutrient-drug interaction
➤ Herbal/supplements-drug interactions.

Table 3.13 Selected food-drug interactions and their clinical implication

Food	Medicine	Type of effect	Clinical Implications
Milk or milk products	Antibiotics Ciprofloxacin Levofloxacin	These antibiotics may bind to the calcium in milk, forming an insoluble substance in the stomach and upper small intestine that the body is unable to absorb. Calcium in the food may decrease the absorption of drugs.	Administer 2 h before or 2 h after milk or milk products.
Grapefruit and grapefruit juice	Cholesterol-lowering drugs(statins) Blood pressure-lowering drugs (Calcium channel blockers nifedipine verapamil) Estrogen containing contraceptives	Grapefruit contains a compound furanocoumarin that inhibits a common drug-metabolizing enzyme called CYP3A4 present in the liver and small intestine Drinking a lot of the juice or eating the fruit inhibits this enzyme, and the drug accumulates in the body. It reduces the metabolism of drugs and increases the risk of side effects.	Avoid grapefruit or grapefruit juice 2 h before or 1 hour.
Apple Juice and Orange juice	Antihistaminic drug(Fexofenadine)	Compete with the absorption of Fexofenadine. Increased absorption by decreased first-pass metabolism can slow heart rate and lower blood pressure.	
Aged cheese, Pickles, yeast extracts, fermented food	Antidepressants Monoamine oxidase inhibitors; Isocarboxazid Phenelzine	Tyramine is naturally found in protein-containing foods. With food aging, the level of tyramine increases. A high level of tyramine causes a sudden, dangerous increase in blood pressure,	Avoid foods and beverages containing tyramine or tryptophan while taking medications and for 2 weeks after stopping this drug.

Table 3.13 *Contd....*

		Normally any ingested amount of tyramine is rapidly broken down in our intestine and liver. When the enzyme activity is inhibited, there could be a potentially fatal rise in blood pressure.	
High-fiber products, such as bran, pectin, bulk laxatives	Cardiac glycosides(Digoxin)	Decreases absorption of the drug.	Administer before 1 hour or 4 h after ingestion of high fiber food products.
Regular meal or snack	Anti-tuberculosis; Rifampin, Rifadin,	Delays or decreases absorption of the drug.	Administer 1 hour before or 2 h after meal or snack.
Soybean formulas	Thyroid supplements	Decreases absorption; increases fecal elimination.	Avoid soybean formulas and Limit foods high in iodine like soybeans, or turnips.
Alcohol	Pain reliever Antihistamines	Liver toxicity Drowsiness	Avoid alcohol

Nutrient–Drug Interactions: Nutrient-drug interactions take place when the nutrient in the consumed food gives an effect on the medication. Factors such as the timing of medication intake and the type of food taken shall be monitored to prevent harmful effects.

Table 3.14 Selected nutrient-drug interactions and their clinical implication

Nutrient in food	Medicine	Type of effect	Clinical implications
Calcium	Ciprofloxacin	Calcium binds with these drugs inhibiting the absorption of the drugs.	Hold enteral feeding 1 hour before and 2 h after administration of the drug.
Potassium	Diuretics, thiazide; Chlorthalidone	Causes loss of potassium and magnesium; can cause rapid heart rate and arrhythmias.	Administer potassium/magnesium supplements or foods such as apricots, bananas, cantaloupe, dairy foods, dried beans, lentils, oranges, and tomatoes.

Table 3.14 *Contd....*

Vitamin D supplements	Gastrointestinal Medications	Calcium toxicity and kidney failure.	Avoid milk; milk products and calcium supplement
Aluminium	Levofloxacin	Aluminum binds with these drugs inhibiting the absorption of the drugs.	Avoid meals that contain aluminum and aluminum supplement.
Iron	Norfloxacin	Iron binds with this drug inhibiting the absorption of the drugs	Avoid meals that contain iron and iron supplement.
Zinc		Zinc binds with the drug inhibiting the absorption of the drugs.	Avoid meals that contain zinc and zinc supplement.
Vitamin K	warfarin	Vitamin K is vital for the production of clotting factors that help prevent bleeding.	Limit foods high in vitamin K such as broccoli, spinach, and turnip greens.
Iodine	Metformin	Decreases absorption; increases fecal elimination	Limit foods high in iodine, such as sprouts, cabbage, soybeans.

Drug-Herb/supplement Interaction: The herbs which we commonly use in our daily food can affect the processing of drugs inside the body and sometimes can lead to serious problems.

Table 3.15 Selected herb/supplement-drug interactions and their clinical implication

Herb/Supplement	Medicine	Type of effect
Garlic	Isoniazid	Reduced absorption of isoniazid
Ginseng	Antihypertensive	Increase in blood pressure
Green tea	Calcium	Decrease calcium absorption
Turmeric	NSAID	Increased gastric irritation bleeding.
Ginger	Warfarin	Increased effectiveness, leads to bleeding
Neem	Insulin	Decrease glucose level

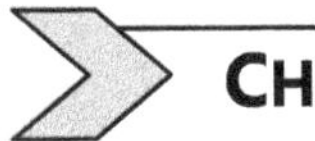 **CHAPTER 4**

Introduction to Microbiology and Common Microorganisms

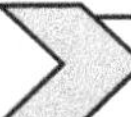 ## 4.1 Microbiology

The word "microbiology" comes from three Greek words (Micro: very small to be seen by the naked eye; Bio: Life; Logy: Science).

> Microbiology is the scientific study of microscopic living organisms such as bacteria, fungi, algae, protozoa, and viruses. Each type has a characteristic cellular composition, morphology, physiology, metabolism, and reproduction.

> There is a close relationship between microbes and human health and well-being. This relationship has helped the host in the metabolism of indigestible substances, supply of important nutrients, protection against specific bacteria, and digestion of certain foods. On the other hand, microorganisms play a role in the development of a variety of diseases, including liver disease, infection, gastric cancer, metabolic issues, respiratory disease, etc.

LEARNING OBJECTIVES

- ♦ Introduction to Microbiology and common microorganisms
- ♦ Epidemiology and its applications.
- ♦ Causative agents, epidemiology and clinical presentations, and the role of Pharmacists in educating the public in the prevention of communicable diseases:
- ♦ **Respiratory infections –** chickenpox, measles, rubella, mumps, influenza (including Avian-Flu, H1N1, SARS, MERS, COVID-19), diphtheria, whooping cough, meningococcal meningitis tuberculosis, Ebola
- ♦ **Intestinal infections –** poliomyelitis, viral hepatitis, cholera, acute diarrheal diseases, typhoid, amoebiasis, worm infestations, food poisoning
- ♦ **Arthropod-borne infections -** dengue, malaria, filariasis, and, chikungunya
- ♦ **Surface infections –** trachoma, tetanus, leprosy
- ♦ STDs, HIV/AIDS

> As a result, Microbiology is now one of the most important biological sciences in our society.

Important characteristics of microorganisms: In order to classify and identify microbes, it is important to understand their characteristics. It is usually impossible to study the characteristics of a single microorganism due to its small size so the properties of a culture containing multiple bacteria of just one type are studied. Different types are based upon:

Morphological characteristics: These include cell arrangement, shape, size, structure, staining, motility, and flagella arrangement. The study of morphological features requires the use of a high-power microscope usually at a magnification of about a thousand times. Depending upon the cellular structure, the microorganisms can be classified into 3 broad groups:

> **Prokaryotic** ("without nucleus"): It is a type of cell that does not have a true nucleus or internal membrane-bound organelles. Organisms include bacteria

> **Eukaryotic** ("true nucleus"): The cells have internal membrane-bound structures (nucleus and organelles) include organisms such as protozoans, fungi, algae, animals, plants

> **Viruses** are acellular: without a cell

Chemical composition: Microbial cells consist of a variety of chemical constituents. Each kind of microorganism is found to have a characteristic chemical composition e.g. cell walls of gram-negative bacteria contain lipopolysaccharide which is not present in the cell wall of gram-positive bacteria.

Cultural characteristics: Different microorganisms require different nutrients and environmental conditions for growth. Some bacteria can grow in a medium with only inorganic components, whereas others require a medium including organic compounds (amino acids, sugars, vitamins).

In addition to different needs for specific nutrients, microbes have varying needs for physical factors such as temperature, light, and oxygen. Microbial diversity is characterized by the following factors:

> **Metabolic characteristics:** The life processes of different microbial cells differ based on how they get and use energy, carry out chemical reactions, and regulate numerous processes. The various chemical reactions of any organism are catalyzed by proteins called enzymes, and the way these enzymes are regulated varies significantly between organisms.

> **Genetic characteristics:** The double-stranded chromosomal DNA of each kind of microorganism has certain features that are constant and characteristics of that organism.

> **Ecological Characteristics:** The habitat of a microorganism is an important characteristic of certain microbial species e.g. microbial population of the oral cavity differs from that of the intestinal tract.

> **Antigenic characteristics:** Antigens are special large chemical components of the bacterial cell and they are distinctive to certain kinds

of microorganisms. After the invasion, the bacteria induce the production of specific antibodies in the host. A single bacterium may carry several antigens which are classified according to the position occupied by them. For example:

- Flagellar antigens are present on the flagella.

- Surface antigens are associated with structures on the surface of the cell.

Antigenic response: When a microbe enters the animal body, the animal responds to these antigens by forming specific blood serum proteins called antibodies which bind to antigens. Antibodies are highly specific to antigens. As different microorganisms have different antigens so antibodies produced in response to that antigen may be used as tools for the rapid identification of specific kinds of organisms.

Microorganisms

Microorganisms may be **single-celled** like bacteria, and protozoa, or **multicellular**, such as algae and fungi.

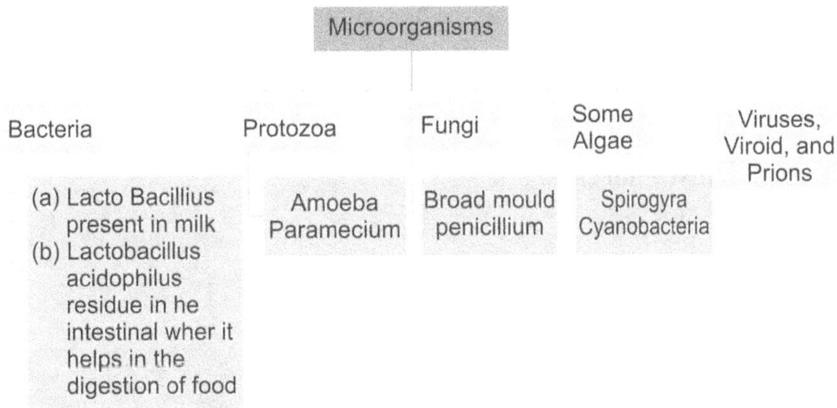

Figure 4.1 Various microorganisms

Diseases caused by various microorganisms: Disease and decomposition are neither basic qualities of the organisms nor the result of physical harm; rather, microbes are responsible for these changes. Numerous microorganisms are known to infect humans and cause a variety of diseases.

Bacteria (study of bacteria – **bacteriology**)

Characteristics

➢ Prokaryotes

➢ Unicellular

➤ Shapes: **bacillus** (rod), **coccus** (spherical), **spirillum** (spiral), **vibrio** (curved rods)

➤ motile or non-motile

Classification: Depending on their requirements and the source of energy use they are classified into different nutritional groups. These are:

➤ **Photosynthetic autotrophs** - use energy from the Sun to produce their own carbohydrates for energy.

➤ **Chemosynthetic autotrophs** - process inorganic molecules for energy (e.g. sulfur or iron).

➤ **Heterotrophs** - depend on outside sources of organic molecules like carbohydrates or sugars for energy.

Viruses - (study of viruses – **virology**)

➤ Acellular, so not considered prokaryotic or eukaryotic.

➤ Obligate intracellular parasites (cannot complete their lifecycle without a host).

➤ The basic structure of a virus - a piece of nucleic acid (RNA or DNA) enclosed by a protein coat (capsid); possesses no nucleus, organelles, cell membrane, or cytoplasm.

➤ Size - 1/10 to 1/1000 is the size of an ordinary bacterial cell.

➤ Non-motile

Protozoa ("first animals")

➤ Eukaryotes

➤ Unicellular

➤ Motile or Non-motile

➤ Heterotrophs

Fungi - (study of fungi – **Mycology**)

➤ Eukaryotic

➤ Unicellular or multicellular (yeasts are unicellular, molds are multicellular).

➤ Non-motile

➤ Heterotrophs

Identification of Microorganisms: Microorganisms are all around and can be identified by different techniques:

➤ **Light microscopy**: Bacteria are too small to be observed by the naked eye so a magnifying microscope is used. Most bacteria are seen with 1000 magnification.

➤ **Gram Staining:** Bacteria are first stained with a weakly alkaline solution of crystal violet or gentian violet. The blue-colored bacteria are treated with a 0.5% iodine solution followed by washing with water and then absolute alcohol. Bacteria stained by the gram method fall into two categories:

➤ **Gram Positive:** They retain the stain and appear deep violet in color e.g. *Streptococcus, Bacillus, Mycobacterium.*

➤ **Gram Negative:** They lose the stain and appear red in color e.g *Vibrio, Salmonella, Pseudomonas,*

Table 4.1 Some important diseases caused by Bacteria, Viruses, Fungi, and Protozoa

Disease	Causative agents	Mode of transmission	Host	Details
Common diseases caused by Bacteria				
Acne/ pimples	Propionibacterium acnes *Acne vulgaris*	Direct contact/close contact	Humans/ Adolescents	Skin disease occurs when hair follicles become clogged with dead skin cells and oil from the skin.
Anthrax	*Bacillus anthrax*	Contact with infected meat	Animals/ Humans	Causes skin infections and Gastrointestinal infections
Cholera	*Vibrio cholerae*	Water/food	Humans	Effects on the small intestine. Severe diarrhea, vomiting, and muscle cramps may also occur.
Diptheria	*Corynebacterium diphtheriae*	Air/direct contact	Humans	Sore throat and fever. The neck may swell in part due to large lymph nodes.
Pneumonia	*Streptococcus pneumoniae* and *Haemophilus influenzae*	Air-borne droplets of sneeze	Humans	Pneumonia is an inflammatory condition of the lung affecting primarily the microscopic air sacs known as alveoli.

Table 4.1 *Contd....*

Disease	Causative agents	Mode of transmission	Host	Details
Peptic ulcers	*Helicobacter pylori*		Humans	Ulcers in the lining of the stomach and starting part of the small intestine.
Tuberculosis	*Mycobacterium tuberculosis*	Air	Humans	Generally affects the lungs
Typhoid	*Salmonella typhi*	Water	Humans	High fever, weakness, abdominal cramps
Common diseases caused by Virus				
AIDS	Human Immunodeficiency Virus (HIV)	Blood exchange	Humans and primates	Severely weakens immunity
Chicken Pox	Varicella Zoster Virus (VZV)	Air/Contact	Humans	Characteristic skin rash that forms small, itchy blisters
Chikungunya	Chikungunya virus	Aedes mosquitoes		Causes severe joint pains.
Influenza	Rhinoviruses	Droplet transmission	Humans	high fever, headache, vomiting, muscle, and joint pains, and a characteristic skin rash.
Dengue fever		Female Aedes mosquito	Humans	low levels of blood platelets and blood plasma leakage.
Ebola	Ebola virus	Animal to man	Humans and Some Animals	lethargy, nausea, diarrhea, and headache
Hepatitis B	hepatitis B virus (HBV)	Blood transfusion, sexual contact	Humans	Affects the **liver**. Acute as well as chronic.
Polio	Poliovirus	Feacal-oral transmission	Humans	Weak muscles lead to deformations.

Table 4.1 *Contd....*

Disease	Causative agents	Mode of transmission	Host	Details
Common diseases caused by Protozoa				
Amoebiasis (amoebic dysentery)	*Entamoeba histolytica*	Contaminated Water/food	Humans	Abdominal pain, mild diarrhoea, bloody diarrhea, or severe colitis with tissue death.
Malaria	Different species of Plasmodium	Female Anopheles mosquito	Humans	Fever, fatigue, vomiting, and headache.
Common diseases caused by fungi				
Ringworms	*Trichophyton, microsporum*	Skin to skin contact	Humans	Fungi feed on keratin, the material found in the outer layer of skin, hair, and nails.
Candidiasis	*Candida albicans*	Skin to skin contact	Humans	Affects skin mucous membranes.

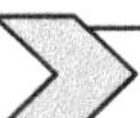

4.2   Introduction of Epidemiology

Epidemiology is a term used to describe the study of disease. It is derived from the word epidemic (epi=among, demos=people; logos=study). **Epidemiology is the basic science of preventive and social medicine.**

Definition: Epidemiology is the study of the frequency, distribution, and determinants of diseases and other health-related conditions in human populations, and the application of this study to the promotion of health and to the prevention and control of health problems.

Concept of Epidemiology: The term "epidemiology" constitutes three components:

1. **Disease frequency**: Epidemiology" is a quantitative science. It provides information about the occurrence of illness is measured in the form of rates and ratios (e.g. prevalence rate, incidence rate, death rate, etc.).

   Epidemiology is also concerned with the measurement of health-related events and states in the community (e.g., health needs, demands, activities, tasks, and health care utilization) and variables such as blood pressure, serum cholesterol, height, weight, etc.

2. **Distribution of disease:** In epidemiology, distribution refers to the occurrence of disease in relation to place, person, and time.

3. **Determinants of disease:** Epidemiology identifies the underlying causes or risk factors of disease. The determinants are factors that determine whether or not a person will get a disease.

Goals of Epidemiology: The ultimate aim of epidemiology is to eliminate or decrease health issues or their effects in order to improve society's health and well-being. According to the International Epidemiological Association (IEA), epidemiology has three main goals:

➢ To describe the **distribution and magnitude** of health and disease problems in human populations (descriptive studies).

➢ To **identify etiological factors** (risk factors) of a disease.

➢ To provide data necessary for the **planning, implementation, and evaluation** of services for disease prevention, control, and treatment (analytical studies).

Uses of Epidemiology: There are seven major uses/applications of epidemiology:

1. **Evaluates the rise and fall of disease in the population:** The pattern of health and disease in a community is never consistent. It varies with time. Epidemiology provides a means to study disease profiles and the time trends in a population. Based on these trends, the future emergence of the disease can be predicted, allowing for necessary actions to be taken.

2. **Community Diagnosis:** The identification and measurement of health concerns in a community in terms of mortality and morbidity rates and ratios are referred to as community diagnosis. It aids in the identification of at-risk individuals or groups, as well as those in need of medical attention.

3. **Health-care planning and evaluation:** Epidemiological information regarding the distribution of health problems over time and place is used to plan, implement, and evaluate health services. It also evaluates the effectiveness of measures to control or prevent a disease, to determine if it reduces disease frequency.

4. **Evaluation of individual risks and chances:** One of the important responsibilities of epidemiologists is to predict the degree of risk in a population

5. **Identification of syndromes:** A number of medical syndromes have been identified as a result of commonly occurring symptoms in individual patients. Epidemiological studies are used to correctly define such syndromes.

6. **Completing the disease's natural history:** In epidemiology, disease trends in the community are investigated in connection to the agent, host, and environmental factors. This clarifies a disease's natural history.

7. **Identifying causes and risk factors of the disease:** Epidemiology helps to identify causes and risk factors of a diswease.

Important Terms in Epidemiology

➢ **Epidemic:** The incidence of any health-related problem in a population at a rate that is greater than the normal frequency of the population.

➢ **Endemic:** It refers to the occurrence of a disease or infectious agent in a certain geographic area or population group on a regular basis e.g. common cold.

➢ **Sporadic:** A disease that only occurs at irregular and frequent intervals in a group of populations e.g. plague, tetanus, and rabies.

➢ **Pandemic**: A disease that has spread across numerous countries and has affected a huge number of people e.g., Covid-19.

➢ **Exotic:** Diseases that are imported into a place where they do not naturally occur, such as rabies in the United Kingdom.

➢ **Zoonosis**: It is an infection or infectious disease that can be transmitted from vertebrate animals to humans in natural situations eg. Rabies, plague, TB, anthrax, etc.

➢ **Epizootic:** An outbreak (epidemic) of disease in an animal population e.g. anthrax, rabies.

➢ **Enzootic:** An endemic disease found only in animals, such as anthrax or rabies.

➢ **Contamination**: It is defined as the presence of an infectious agent on items such as clothing, bedding, toys, surgical equipment, or bandages, as well as substances such as water, milk, and food.

➢ **Infestation**: It is defined as the presence of a living infectious agent on the body's outer surface.

➢ **Infection**: The growth of an infectious agent in the body of a person or animal is called an infection.

➢ **Infectious agents:** Any agents that can cause infection.

➢ **Infectious disease**: A disease that manifests clinically in humans or animals as a result of an infection.

➢ **Contagious disease:** A disease that is transmitted through contact e.g. scabies, trachoma, leprosy.

➢ **Nosocomial infection:** It is an infection contacted by a patient while visiting or staying in a hospital or other healthcare institution.

➢ **Eradication:** It means the termination of an infection from the whole world. It implies that the disease will no longer occur in a population.

➢ **Surveillance**: It is the continuous examination of the factors that determine the occurrence and distribution of disease and other conditions of ill health.

➢ **Quarantine:** It refers to restricting the movement of people who may have been exposed to a contagious disease but have no confirmed diagnosis. The quarantine period equals the maximum incubation period of the disease.

➢ **Isolation:** Medical isolation is imposed only after a confirmed diagnosis of a communicable disease. Isolation separates sick /infected people from people who are not sick.

➢ **Incubation period:** In medicine, the interval between exposure to an infectious agent and the appearance of signs and symptoms of the disease is known as the incubation period. Chicken pox, for example, takes 14-16 days to incubate.

➢ **Contact tracing:** It is a method of identifying and notifying those who have been exposed to an infectious disease. It is carried out in order to control the number of infections in the community. It includes tracing the contacts of infected individuals, testing them for infection, and isolating or treating the infected e.g. Covid-19, Ebola, H1N1.

➢ The goals of contact tracing are:

- To stop an infection from spreading further.

- To warn contacts about the risk of infection and provide preventive services or prophylactic care.

- To provide diagnosis, counseling, and treatment to already infected individuals.

- To help prevent re-infection of the originally infected patient, if the infection is treatable.

- To learn about the epidemiology of a disease in a specific population.

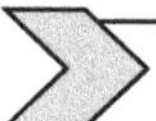

4.3   Communicable Diseases

A communicable disease is one that is caused by a specific infectious agent or its toxic products, and can be transmitted from person to person, animal to animal, or from the environment (air, dust, soil, water, food) to man or animal.

A.   Disease Transmission:

In the chain of disease transmission and the spread of the disease, the following six factors are involved:

    I. **Causative Agent:** The microorganism capable of causing an infection (for example bacteria, virus or fungi, protozoa, metazoan, etc).

    II. **Source (Reservoir) of infection:** It is any person, animal, arthropod, plant, substance, soil, or environment in which an infectious agent survives and multiplies before infecting a susceptible host.

III. Portal of Exit: A path for the microorganism to escape from the host. Microorganisms escape through blood, lungs, skin, mucosal membranes, the genitourinary system, GI tract, and trans placental pathways.

IV. Mode of Transmission - The mechanisms by which an infectious agent is transferred from one person to another or from a reservoir to a new host. Infectious agents from a reservoir or source can be transferred in several ways.

    a)   Direct Transmission:

- **Direct Contact**: This involves transferring an infectious agent from its source or reservoir to a susceptible person. e.g. touching, kissing, or sexual relations. HIV, leprosy, conjunctivitis, and skin infections.

- **Droplet Infection**: Minute droplets of saliva and nasopharyngeal secretions are released into the atmosphere during sneezing, coughing, spitting, singing, and talking, When individuals inhale these infectious droplets, some of them get infected e.g. common cold, diphtheria, whooping cough, and tuberculosis.

- **Contact with soil:** Direct exposure to an infectious agent in soil, compost, or decomposing vegetable waste can cause infections like hookworm, tetanus, mycosis, etc.

- **Bite of an animal:** It can lead to direct transmission of disease e.g. rabies.

- **Trans placental transmission:** Certain diseases are transmitted through the placenta e.g. syphilis, hepatitis B, and AIDS.

    b)   Indirect Transmission

- **Vehicle-borne transmission:** Infectious agents spread through contaminated water, food, ice, blood, serum, plasma, or other biological products. Common diseases are diarrhea, typhoid, cholera, hepatitis A, food poisoning, and intestinal parasites.

- **Vector-borne transmission:** Vector is an arthropod or any living carrier that transports an infectious agent to a susceptible individual e.g. transmission of malaria by mosquitos, plague by rats, cholera by the house fly.

- **Air-borne transmission:** Microbial agents transfer to the respiratory tract through the air. Dust and droplet nuclei are two types of particles involved in this form of diffusion.

- **Dust**: microscopic infectious particles suspended by air from dirt, clothes, bedding, or contaminated floors.
- **Droplet nuclei**: Small residues usually remain suspended for a longer time in the air. Pneumonia, TB, streptococcal, and hospital-acquired infections are among the diseases spread by dust and droplets.
- **Fomite-borne transmission**: Contaminated clothes, towels, linen, handkerchiefs, pencils, books, toys, drinking glasses, taps, lavatory chains, and door knobs can spread an infectious agent.
- **Poor hygiene**: Poor sanitation and personal hygiene favor the spread of infection from person to person. Staphylococcal, typhoid, dysentery, hepatitis, and intestinal parasites are a few examples.

V. **Portal of Entry:** A path for the microorganism to get into a new host, similar to the portal of exit.

VI. **Susceptible host (host factors):** A person that lacks sufficient resistance to a certain pathogenic agent is referred to as a susceptible host. Host factors influence both the occurrence of infection and its outcome. The capacity of the host to fight infection is referred to as "immunity."

Time course of Disease:

➤ **Incubation Period:** It is the interval of time between infection of the host and the first appearance of signs and symptoms of the disease.

➤ **Prodromal period:** The period that precedes the onset of symptoms.

➤ **Period of communicability**: The time period in which an infectious agent can be transferred from an infected person to a susceptible person.

B. **Disease Prevention**: There are three levels of disease prevention: primary, secondary, and tertiary.

Primary prevention: It is done before the onset of the disease with the objective *to promote health, prevent exposure, and prevent disease.*

➤ *Health promotion:* Health promotion measures are aimed at increasing socioeconomic status by providing well-paid jobs, education, vocational training, housing, clothing, food, old-age pensions, emotional and social support, etc.

➤ *Prevention of exposure*: This includes actions such as the provision of safe and adequate water, proper excreta disposal, vector control, and a safe environment at home.

➤ *Prevention of disease*: Immunization is one of the important methods to protect the organism from developing an infection.

Secondary prevention: It is done after the biological onset of disease, but before permanent damage sets in. Its objective is *to stop or slow the progression of the disease to prevent permanent damage* e.g. early detection and treatment of breast cancer prevent the advanced phase of the disease.

Tertiary prevention: It may be done after permanent damage has set in. Its objective is *to limit the impact of that damage.*

C. **Communicable Disease Control:** This refers to the reduction of the incidence and prevalence of communicable diseases to a level where it cannot be a major public health problem. There are three main methods of controlling communicable diseases:

(i) *Elimination of the Reservoir: When a man is a reservoir, the following measures can be taken:*

> Breaking the communicability of the disease **by detection and adequate treatment** of cases e.g. in case of treatment of Covid-19.

> **Isolation:** Separation of infected persons for a period of communicability of the disease.

> **Quarantine:** Movement restriction for a person exposed to the infectious disease for the maximal incubation time.

In the case of animals as reservoirs action must be based on their relationship to man, and the possibility of saving animal species. For example:

> **Plague:** The rat is regarded as a pest and the objective would be to destroy the rat and exclude it from human habitation.

> **Rabies:** Dogs can be protected by vaccination.

> Infected animals used for food are examined and destroyed.

In the case the reservoir is a non-living thing: Limit man's exposure to the affected area (e.g., soil, water, forest, etc.) or use appropriate sanitization and disinfection measures.

The following section of the chapter discusses various causative agents, epidemiology and clinical presentations, and the role of pharmacists in educating the public in the prevention of communicable diseases viz **Respiratory infections, intestinal infections, Arthropod-borne infections, surface infections, and sexually transmitted infections.**

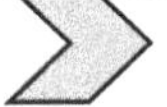

4.4   Respiratory Infections

Respiratory infections are diseases transmitted by infected patients via respiratory discharges like coughs, laughs, sneezes, fluid discharges, and fluid droplets. Fine droplets enter the body via the respiratory tract. Air-borne diseases can spread more easily when there is overcrowding, as in overcrowded public transport, classrooms, and canteens etc.

Chickenpox

Introduction: It is an acute infection and is a highly contagious disease caused by Varicella Zoster Virus (VZV). The infection causes itchy rashes that form small, itchy blisters, which eventually flake over. Infection gives a long immunity.

Epidemiology: In temperate countries, chickenpox is primarily a disease of children, with most cases occurring during the winter and spring, most likely due to school contact.

Table 4.2 General characteristic features of Chickenpox

Chickenpox	
Infectious agent:	**Varicella Zoster Virus**
Reservoir	Humans
Incubation period	14 to 16 days
Susceptibility and resistance	Children under age 2 are at most risk for chicken pox.
Period of communicability	Communicable 5 days before the rash appear and up to 5 days after onset of lesions.

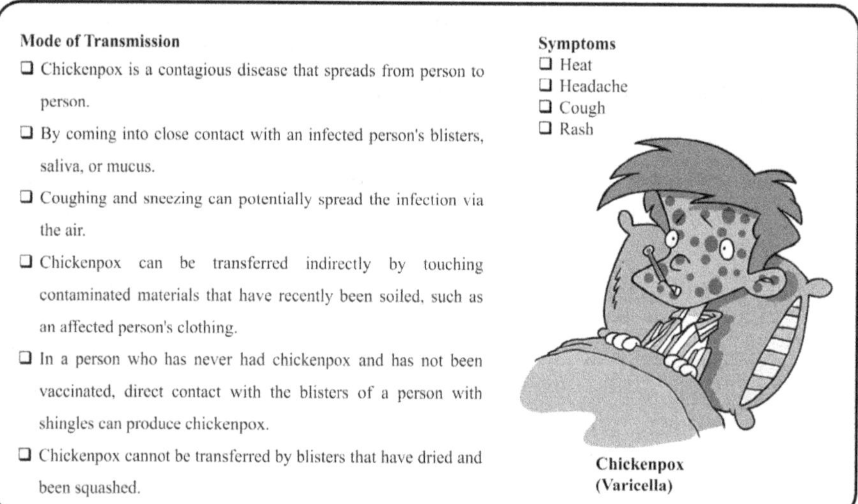

Figure 4.2 Mode of transmission of Chickenpox

Transmission: The disease is transmitted by droplet infection and the virus enters the upper respiratory tract. The discharge from the skin lesions can also infect others. The disease is mild and provides immunity for the rest of life.

Clinical manifestation: The itchy blister rash caused by chickenpox infection appears 10 to 21 days after exposure to the virus and usually lasts about 5 to 10 days. The common symptoms are:

➢ Fever, loss of appetite, and headache.

➢ Tiredness and a general feeling of being unwell (malaise), body aches, dizziness, and dehydration.

Once the chickenpox rash appears, it goes through three phases:

➢ Raised pink or red bumps (**papules**), which break out over several days.

➢ Small fluid-filled blisters (**vesicles**), form in about a day and then leak.

➢ Crusts and scabs **(Pustules),** cover the broken blisters and take several days to heal.

Prevention and control:

➢ The disease can be prevented by educating parents to get their children vaccinated with the chicken pox vaccine as per the immunization schedule.

➢ The spread of infection can be avoided by isolating the patient.

➢ Paracetamol is advised to control fever and pain associated with sores, to relieve itching some local soothing agents may be applied. Pain killers like ibuprofen and aspirin which can lead to a serious complication called Reye's syndrome are contraindicated.

➢ It is important to drink plenty of fluids, preferably water, to prevent dehydration.

Measles

Introduction: Measles is a highly contagious and severe viral disease. Nine out of ten people who are not immune and share a common space with an infected person can become infected.

Epidemiology: Vaccines are effective against measles. Prior to the introduction of vaccines, it was the top cause of death globally among children under the age of five. 90% of people get infected by age 20, and few do not get infection throughout their life. India had the lowest incidence rate for measles.

Table 4.3 General characteristic features of Measles

Measles	
Infectious agent:	***Morbillivirus, Paramyxovirus***
Reservoir	Humans
Incubation period	8 to 14 days
Susceptibility and resistance	Non-vaccinated infants and children below age 5, adults below age 20, and pregnant women are most susceptible.
Period of communicability	Communicable 4 days before the rash appears and up to 4 days after onset of rash.

Transmission: Direct contact with infectious airborne droplets spreads the virus. The virus is transmitted when an infected person breathes, coughs, or sneezes.

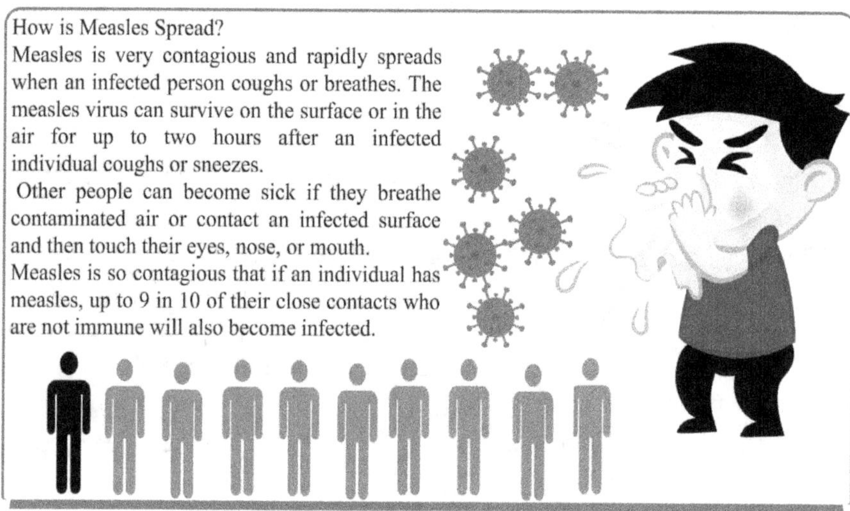

Figure 4.3 Transmission of measles

Clinical manifestations: Most common symptoms are:

➤ Elevation in body temperature (hyperpyrexia; 104°F).

➤ Runny nose (coryza).

➤ The appearance of red spots in the mouth (Koplik's spots).

➤ A sudden, forceful hacking sound, an irritation in the throat and airway.

➤ Red watery eyes with overproduction of tears.

➤ Temporary outbreak of red bumpy, scaly or itchy patches of skin. The macular rash is first seen at the backside of the ears and on the forehead across the hairline then spreads to the whole body. The rash fades from the face downwards in the same sequence as the appearance.

Prevention and control:

➢ Vaccination is the best way to prevent measles. There are two vaccines available for measles: The MMR and MMRV vaccine. (Provision of measles vaccine at nine months of age).

➢ Educate the public about measles immunization.

➢ Wear masks and follow hygiene etiquettes (practice good hand hygiene. wash your hands before eating, after using the bathroom, and before touching your face, mouth, or nose)

➢ Prevent contact with the infected person

Rubella

Introduction: Rubella (German measles) is also known as three-day measles. It is a mild infection caused by the rubella virus.

Congenital rubella: This is a condition that defines infants born to rubella-infected mothers during the first trimester of pregnancy. The risk of congenital abnormalities is dependent on when the infection occurs during pregnancy. Rubella infection during the first few weeks of pregnancy increases the chance of different fetal abnormalities, but infection throughout the third trimester of pregnancy has little risk.

Epidemiology: In India, 40-45% of childbearing women are susceptible to rubella infection. Over 2 lakh babies are born with a birth defect because of rubella infection during pregnancy in the Indian subcontinent.

Table 4.4 General characteristic features of Rubella

Rubella (German measles)	
Infectious agent:	*Rubella virus*
Reservoir	Humans are the only reservoir
Incubation period	16-18 days; range 14-23 days.
Susceptibility and resistance	Children, young adults, and pregnant women are most common in primary school children. Vaccinated children and adults are resistant.
Period of communicability	1 week before to 5-7 days after onset of rash.

Transmission: The virus may be transmitted from person to person via direct or droplet contact from nasopharyngeal secretions, through urine, and trans-placental transmission occurs from mother to fetus.

Clinical manifestation: Symptoms that often appear two to three weeks after exposure to rubella virus include:

➢ Mild pyrexia may occur 24 hours before the appearance of the rash. For 1-2 days, there may be mild malaise and painful lymph nodes behind the ears and the back of the head. Arthritis of the hands or feet can affect older children or adults.

➢ The pink or red macular rash begins on the face and then spreads downwards to the rest of the body.

➢ Reddening of eyes, inflammation around the eyes, runny eyes, and sharp to dull headache, soreness and muscle pain.

➢ Excess secretions ranging from a clear fluid to thick mucus from the nose and nasal passage.

Clinical Manifestations of congenital rubella: Congenital defects of the heart, eyes, and ears, an enlarged liver and spleen, and marked thrombocytopenia (absence of platelets in the blood) are common.

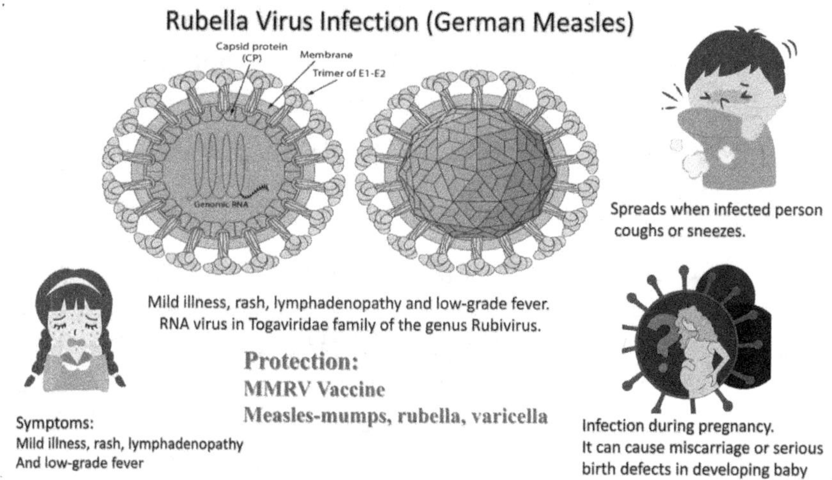

Figure 4.4 Rubella Virus- transmission, common symptoms and prevention

Prevention and Control

➢ **Specific Treatment**: One dose of the rubella virus vaccine gives lifelong immunity.

➢ **Vaccination of children before puberty**: MMR vaccines are given in the second year of life. MMR vaccine is 97% effective at preventing rubella. Girls should be vaccinated before menstruation.

➢ **Avoiding Exposure**: Isolate rubella patient for 7 days after onset of rash. Pregnant women should avoid exposure to the rubella virus.

➤ **Screening and contact tracing**: Rubella antibody test determines the developed immunity in women. Non-immune pregnant women should be vaccinated after delivery. Pregnancy should be avoided within 3 months of receiving the rubella vaccine.

Role of Pharmacist

➤ Health education: Health education about vaccination.

➤ Advising females planning pregnancy to check rubella antibody status.

➤ Health promotion: Manage the treatment of the patient

Mumps

Introduction: Mumps is an acute viral infection that affects the salivary glands, particularly, the parotid gland in 60% of cases; therefore is also called "infectious parotitis". Mumps is characterized by puffy cheeks and a swollen jaw. The virus can travel through the bloodstream to organs and the CNS. Mumps causes puffy cheeks and a swollen jaw.

Epidemiology: Patients of mumps are found worldwide and nearly 50% of infections are asymptomatic. In the absence of vaccination against mumps, there are between 100 and 1,000 active cases per 100,000 people each year. The highest number of cases are found in children 5–9 years old. Cases usually occur in winter and spring. In India, outbreaks are reported throughout the year from all regions of the country.

Table 4.5 General characteristic features of Mumps

Mumps	
Infectious agent:	*Paramyxovirus*
Reservoir	Humans are the only reservoir.
Incubation period	12–28 days, usually about 18 days
Susceptibility and resistance	Children aged between 4–14 years and unvaccinated adults are most commonly affected. Vaccinated children and adults are resistant.
Period of communicability	From 1–3 days before the facial swelling is apparent to about 7 days after the swelling has disappeared.

Transmission: Transmission is by airborne droplets spread from the saliva of an infected patient, and by contact with contaminated articles.

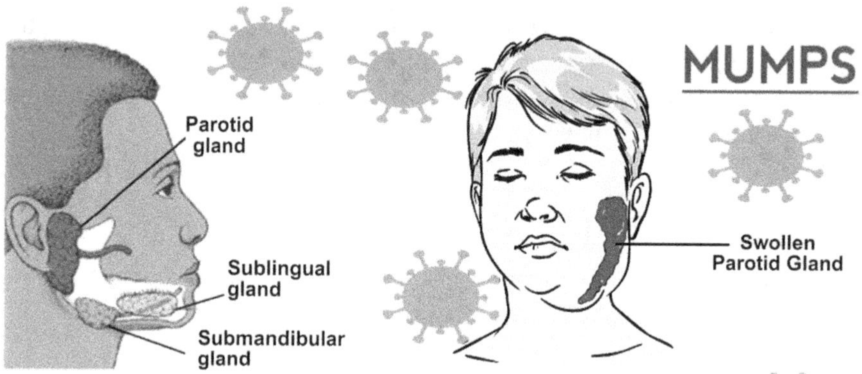

Figure 4.5 Mumps: inflammation of parotid glands

Clinical manifestation

➢ Prodromal symptoms may occur 1 or 2 days before the parotid swelling and are characterized by fever, malaise, and pain behind the ear on chewing or swallowing, or opening the mouth.

➢ As the infection progresses there is a tenderness of the salivary glands for 1-3 days; swelling of the salivary glands for 7–10 days.

➢ Loss of appetite, headache, dizziness, and feeling of fatigue with normal daily activities.

Prevention and Control:

➢ Vaccination provides immunity against mumps infection. The mumps vaccine is usually given as a combined measles-mumps-rubella (MMR) inoculation, which contains the safest and most effective form of each vaccine.

➢ Two doses of MMR vaccine are recommended before a child enters school.

➢ Paracetamol is recommended for fever and muscle pain.

➢ Soothing of swollen glands by applying ice packs.

➢ Drink plenty of fluids to avoid dehydration due to a fever.

Influenza

Introduction: Commonly called Flu, it is an acute disease of the respiratory tract.

Epidemiology: It is prevalent worldwide. The disease could be in form of pandemics, epidemic and there may be a localized outbreak.

Table 4.6 General characteristic features of Influenza

Influenza	
Infectious agent	Influenza virus (A, B and C)
Reservoir	Humans with active disease
Incubation period	1-3 days
Period of communicability	In adults: 3-5 days In young children, up to 7 days after signs of disease appear.
Susceptibility and resistance	When a new sub-type appears, all children and adults are equally susceptible. Infection imparts immunity to the specific infectious agent.

Transmission: The virus enters the body through the respiratory tract. Influenza is transmitted mostly through droplet infection or droplet nuclei formed by speaking, sneezing, or coughing. The virus circulates throughout the year, and outbreaks commonly occur during the winter months. In densely populated areas, such as schools, institutions, railroads, and buses, the prevalence is high.

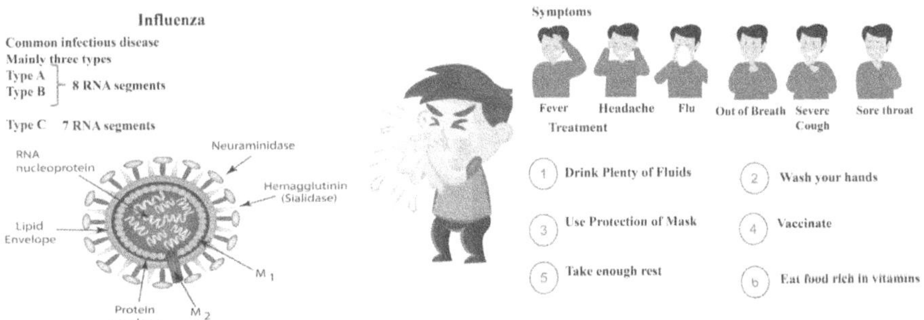

Figure 4.6 Influenza: Symptoms and preventive measures

Clinical manifestations

➢ The virus enters the respiratory tract and causes inflammation and necrosis of the superficial epithelium of the tracheal and bronchial mucosa.

➢ The signs and symptoms include headache, myalgia, fever, sore throat, and cough.

➢ The recovery is in within 2-7days.

Prevention and Control

➢ Immunization with available vaccines that may provide 70-80% protection from the disease.

➢ Educating people on the proper way to cough and sneeze.

➢ Educating the public on fundamental personal hygiene.

➢ Avoiding crowded areas during an epidemic.

➢ At the first sign of influenza, sufferers should be advised to stay at home.

➢ Two neuraminidase inhibitors (Zanamivir, and Oseltamivir) are available for prophylaxis and treatment of influenza A and B.

➢ The sufferers should be advised to stay at home at the first sign of influenza.

H1N1 (Swine Flu)

Swine flu is a respiratory infection caused by the influenza A virus. The disease is known as swine flu because the causative viruses are structurally similar to viruses that infect pigs. H1N1 is a virus composed of swine, avian (bird), and human DNA that mutated in pigs and spread to people. H1N1 is now recognized as a common type of seasonal flu and is included in flu vaccines.

Epidemiology: In 2009–2010, there was a worldwide outbreak, and deaths from the swine flu pandemic reached 575,400.

Table 4.7 General characteristic features of Swine Flu

Swine flu H1N1	
Infectious agent:	*H1N1 strain of influenza virus*
Reservoir	Humans
Incubation period	1-3 days
Susceptibility and resistance	Children under the age of five, pregnant women, and people above 65 years are the most affected. Vaccinated children and adults are resistant.
Period of communicability	From 1-5 days before the symptoms develop, and remain contagious for a longer time.

Transmission: Inhaling infected droplets spread the disease. Swine flu does not spread through the consumption of cooked pork, although it can pass from pigs to humans in pig ponds and livestock farms.

Clinical manifestations: Signs and symptoms include fever, chills, malaise, diarrhoea, vomiting, cough, and sore throat. Throat pain, runny or stuffy nose, red watery eyes, lung infections, body aches, and joint pain or headache.

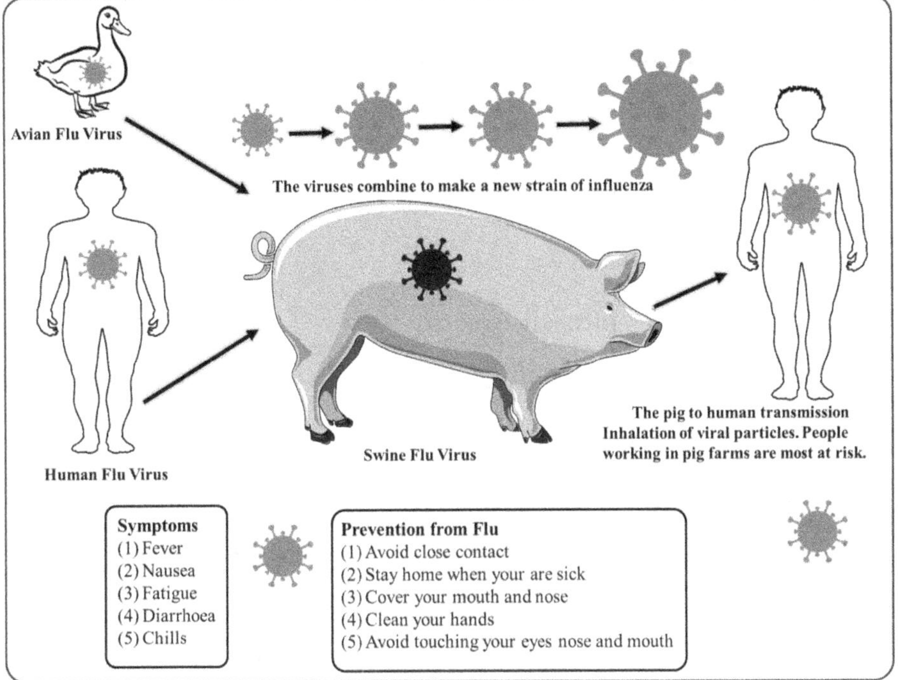

Figure 4.7 Swine flu- transmission, symptoms, and prevention

Prevention and Control

➢ Hands should be washed thoroughly and frequently.

➢ Avoid touching the nose eyes and mouth.

➢ Staying away from crowded places.

➢ Wearing face masks when staying or working outside.

➢ Vaccination: Two types of vaccines are available, killed virus and live virus. These can be given by injections and nasal sprays respectively.

Severe Acute Respiratory Syndrome (SARS)

Severe Acute Respiratory Syndrome (SARS) is an acute viral disease that was first identified in 2003 as a serious form of pneumonia. This zoonotic disease is caused by severe acute respiratory syndrome coronavirus (SARS-CoV or SARS-CoV-1).

Epidemiology: Severe acute respiratory syndrome (SARS) after its origin in Southern China in November 2002 had a worldwide spread mostly to Asian countries. It affected people of all ages but predominantly females. In India, the younger age group was more vulnerable to infection. The global epidemic in 2003 resulted in 916 deaths and the case fatality rate was 11%.

Table 4.8 General characteristic features of SARS

Severe Acute Respiratory Syndrome (SARS)		
Bat Civet SARS-CoV	Infectious agent	Severe acute respiratory syndrome coronavirus (SAR-COV)
	Reservoir	Originated in bats and transmitted to humans via Civet cats (Paguma larvata)
	Incubation period	Around 3 to 10 days
	Period of communicability-	Less than 21 days
	Susceptibility	Young people and females are at more risk.

Transmission: SARS-CoV-1 spread from horseshoe bats to palm civet (cats) hosts and then to humans via cross-infection. In the second week after the beginning of early symptoms, SARS-CoV-1 spreads through respiratory droplets from patients and direct contact or contact with contaminated surfaces.

Clinical manifestations: Symptoms generally appear 2 to 10 days after contracting the virus. The most common are productive cough and runny nose, nausea, vomiting, diarrhoea, muscle aches, headache, persistent fever, respiratory distress or shortness of breath, and reduced respiration capacity.

Prevention:

➤ Avoid direct contact with SARS patients for 10 days after their fever and other symptoms diminish. Avoid sharing food, drinks, or utensils.

➤ Avoid traveling to uncontrollable SARS outbreak areas.

➤ Hand hygiene is key to preventing SARS. Wash or sanitize hands with alcohol.

Middle East Respiratory Syndrome (MERS)

Middle East Respiratory Syndrome (MERS) is a respiratory disease caused by the Middle East Respiratory Syndrome Coronavirusrus, often known as MERS-CoV. This virus was originally detected in Saudi Arabia in 2012. MERS-CoV is a zoonotic virus that most likely originated from an animal source. It has been identified in camels in various countries, in addition to humans. Some people may have become infected after coming into contact with camels.

Epidemiology: About 3 to 4 out of every 10 people infected with MERS had died. Most of the people who died had underlying medical conditions.

Transmission: MERS-CoV, like other coronaviruses, is thought to spread from an infected person's respiratory secretions, such as through coughing. It is transmitted from infected people to others through close contact most likely to the caregivers in hospitals.

Clinical Manifestations: Signs and symptoms include:

➢ Some infected people have mild symptoms like a cold or no symptoms at all.

➢ Some have a severe acute respiratory illness with symptoms of runny nose, sore throat, congestion, shortness of breath, and cough.

➢ Pneumonia and respiratory failure in severe cases.

➢ others symptoms are fever, loss of taste or smell, nausea, and diarrhea.

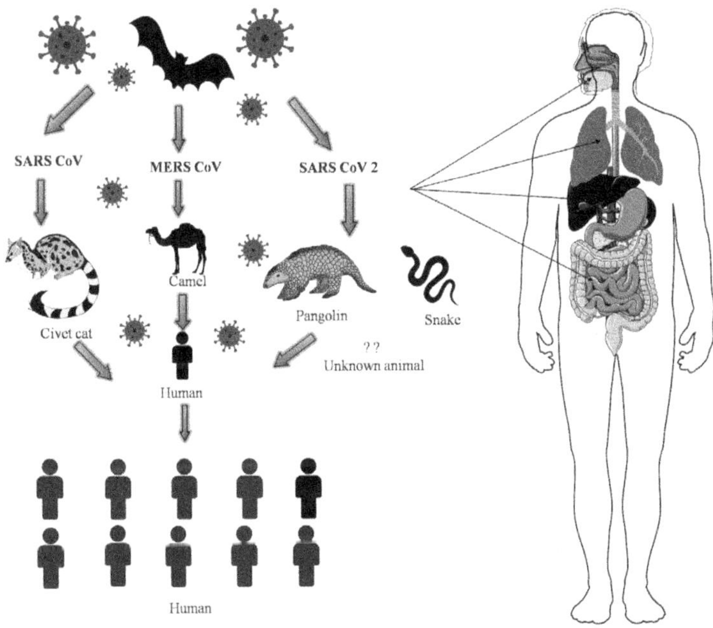

Figure 4.8 Transmission of SARS CoV, MERS CoV, SARS CoV2

Prevention and control:

➢ Wash hands often with soap and water for 20 seconds or uses an alcohol-based hand sanitizer.

➢ Wear masks, maintain social distancing.

➢ Avoid personal contact with sick people.

➢ Disinfect surfaces.

Treatment:

➢ There is currently no vaccine to protect against MERS.

➢ There is no specific antiviral treatment recommended for MERS-CoV infection. Only symptomatic treatment is given.

Covid-19

Coronavirus (COVID-19) is a contagious disease caused by Severe Acute Respiratory Syndrome Coronavirus 2 (SARS-CoV-2). The disease has since spread worldwide, leading to a pandemic.

Epidemiology: First identified in Wuhan, China, in December 2019, the disease has spread globally, infecting over 100 million people and causing over 2 million deaths by March 2021. India reported its first case on 30 January 2020, with 11 million confirmed cases.

Table 4.9 General characteristic features of COVID-19

COVID-19	
Infectious agent	**Coronavirus**
Reservoir	Bats are reservoirs for coronavirus
Incubation period	1 to 14 days
Period of communicability	Less than 21 days
Susceptibility	People of any age but mostly middle-aged and old age people
Resistant	Vaccinated people

Transmission: The virus spreads mainly between people who are in close contact with each other. SARS-CoV-2 transmission can occur via infected secretions such as saliva and respiratory secretions or respiratory droplets expelled when an infected person coughs, sneezes, talks, or sings, or through direct, indirect, or close contact with infected people. This is often called short-range aerosol or short-range airborne transmission.

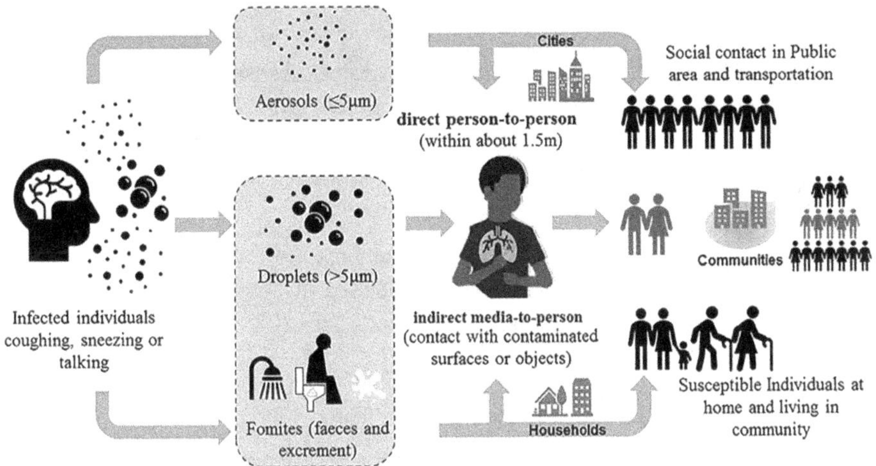

Figure 4.9 Mode of transmission of COVID-19

Clinical manifestations: Most common symptoms include:

➤ Fever, tiredness, headache, muscle aches, loss of taste or smell.

➤ Dyspnea, dry cough sore throat difficulty breathing or shortness of breath, chest pain or pressure.

➤ Diarrhea, conjunctivitis, skin rash, discoloration of fingers or toes.

Prevention and control:

1. Get vaccinated when it's your turn.
2. Isolation of the patients from healthy persons.
3. Case management.
4. Follow sneezing and coughing etiquette. Cover your nose and mouth with your bent elbow or a tissue when you cough or sneeze.
5. Maintain a safe distance from others (at least 1 meter), even if they don't appear to be sick.
6. Wear a mask in public, especially indoors or when social distancing is not feasible.
7. Choose open, well-ventilated spaces over closed ones.
8. Open a window if indoors.
9. Clean your hands often. Use soap and water, or an alcohol-based hand rub.
10. Stay home if you feel unwell. If you have a fever, cough, and difficulty breathing, seek medical advice.

Diphtheria

Introduction: Diphtheria is an acute infectious disease affecting the upper respiratory tract including the throat and caused by the bacteria **Corynebacterium diphtheria**. The disease takes its name from the Greek word diphtheria meaning leather. In this disease, a leathery sheath-like membrane grows on the tonsils, throat, and nose.

Epidemiology: About a million cases a year are believed to have occurred before the 1980s. Now it is an endemic disease in countries like Indonesia, Bangladesh, South Africa, and Myanmar. In 2020, the world's total diphtheria cases were estimated to be 10107.

Table 4.10 General characteristic features of Diphtheria

Infectious agent	*Corynebacterium diphtheria*
Reservoir	Humans and rarely fomites (objects)
Incubation period	2 to 5 days may range up to 10 days.
Period of communicability	Untreated patients are contagious up to 2-6 weeks.
Susceptibility	Unvaccinated individuals.
Resistant	Vaccinated people

Transmission: Human-to-human transmission occurs through oral and respiratory droplets when an infected individual coughs or sneezes. Contact with any lesions/wounds on the skin of an infected person can also lead to transmission of diphtheria. The articles/ objects contaminated with bacteria may also serve as a reservoir of infection.

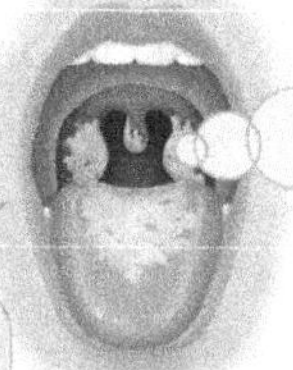

Figure 4.10 Diphtherial sheath over tonsils and throat

Clinical manifestation

➢ A greenish-grey membrane develops over the tonsils and throat. It is generally surrounded by a zone of inflammation. The membrane may obstruct the airway and hence breathing.

➢ Nasal diphtheria symptoms include clear/blood-stained nasal discharge.

➢ Laryngeal diphtheria that spreads from the larynx has symptoms like sore throat, husky voice, high-pitched cough, and danger of respiratory obstruction which can be fatal if tracheotomy is not carried out.

➢ There may be swelling of the neck (bull neck) and tender enlargement of the lymph nodes.

➢ The pulse is weak and rapid and blood pressure is low.

➢ Death from circulatory failure may occur if the condition is not treated within the first 10 days.

Prevention and Control

➢ **Vaccination:** Vaccination is the best way to prevent the disease. The diphtheria vaccine is combined with vaccines for tetanus and whooping cough known as the DPT Vaccine. A total of five shots in a series are given at the age of 2 months--4 months-- 6 months- 15 to 18 month, 4 to 6 years.

➢ **Treatment:** Antibiotics are given to patients or carriers to eradicate C.diphtheriae and prevent its transmission to others.

➢ **Isolation**: the patient/s should be isolated from the healthy children.

➢ **Disinfection:** The articles and clothes used by the patient should be periodically disinfected.

Whooping Cough

Pertussis (whooping cough) is a highly infectious bacterial disease involving the respiratory tract. The causative bacteria are ***Bordetella pertussis*** in more than 90% of cases or rarely ***Bordatella parapertussis.***

Epidemiology: It is an endemic disease common in children, especially young children everywhere in the world. 90% of attacks occur in children under 6 years of age. Out of approximately 20–40 million/year cases of pertussis worldwide each year, 90% occur in developing countries, and approximately, 200 000–300 000 children die of this every year.

Table 4.11 General characteristic features of Whooping Cough

Whooping cough	
Infectious agent	*Bordetella pertussis*
Reservoir	Humans
Incubation period	1-3 weeks
Period of communicability	Non-immunized individuals are susceptible. One attack usually provides prolonged immunity but may not be lifelong.
Susceptibility	From one week before to three weeks after the onset of paroxysmal coughing.

Transmission: The disease is transmitted by the airborne route, primarily by direct contact with discharges from respiratory mucus membranes of infected persons. Indirectly by handling objects contaminated with nasopharyngeal secretions.

Clinical Manifestations: The onset of the disease follows 3 phases:

1. **Catarrhal phase** (Lasts 1-2 weeks): Watery nose and eyes (rhinorrhea), loss of appetite, sneezing, cough, and fever.

2. **Paroxysmal phase (Spasmodic stage)** (Lasts 1-6 weeks):
   - Sudden recurrence of violent and prolonged cough.
   - The child usually vomits at the end of a paroxysm (spasmodic cough).
   - Paroxysm of cough interferes with nutrition.
   - Child looks healthy between paroxysms.
   - Whoop (inspiratory whoop against a closed glottis) between paroxysms.
   - Cyanosis due to apnea (slow breathing), brain damage, and sub conjunctiva hemorrhage due to violent cough.

3. **Convalescent phase (may last for months)**
   - The cough may diminish slowly or may last a long time.
   - After improvement, the disease may recur.

Complications of disease:

Pneumonia, convulsions due to cerebral anoxia during coughing paroxysms; Brain damage as a result of cerebral anoxia; Deafness, and blindness can result from hemorrhages into the conjunctiva during coughing paroxysms; Hernias and rectal prolapse can occur due to repeated coughing.

Prevention and Control:

1. Immunization is the key to prevention.

2. Administer oxygen in severe cases to reduce the severity of cerebral anoxia and the incidence of convulsions and brain damage.

3. Steam inhalations may help those with thick mucus secretions.

4. Small frequent feeds are best given after paroxysmal coughing.

5. Administer antibiotics if secondary bacterial infection occurs. Erythromycin- to treat the infection in phase one and to decrease transmission.

6. Immunization.

Meningococcal Meningitis

Meningococcal meningitis is meningitis due to the bacteria *Neisseria meningitides*. It is an acute bacterial disease that causes inflammation of the pia and arachnoid space.

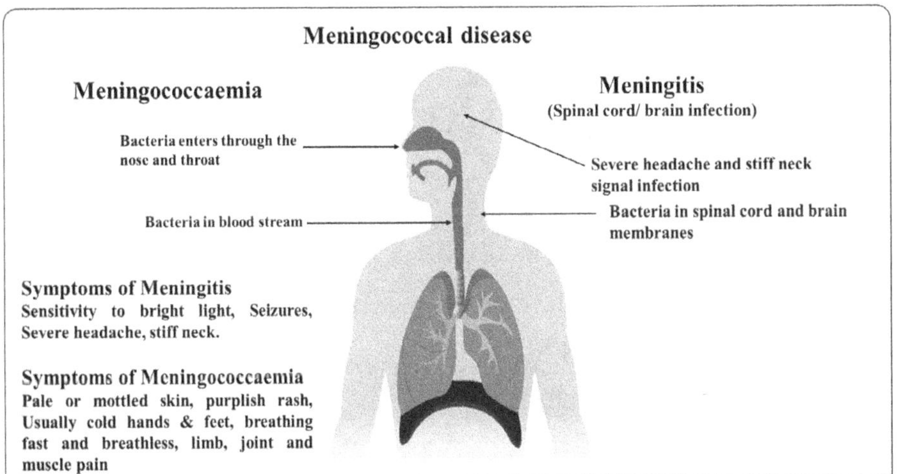

Figure 4.11 Meningitis

Epidemiology: Meningococcal infections occur worldwide and are notifiable in most countries. The greatest incidence occurs during winter and spring. About two-thirds of cases occur in the first 5 years of life. Acute meningitis causes about 150000 deaths per year. Epidemic meningitis due to *Neisseria meningitis* is common in Sub - Saharan Africa and is also seen in parts of Asia. Meningococcal infection is prevalent in India but remains underreported.

Transmission: The bacteria only infect humans and are transmitted from one person to another through droplets of respiratory/ throat/ nasal secretions.

Table 4.12 General characteristic features of Meningococcal infections

Meningococcal meningitides	
Infectious agent	*Neisseria meningitis's*
Reservoir	Humans
Incubation period	2-10 day, commonly 3-4 days
Period of communicability	Susceptibility is low and decreases with age.
Susceptibility	Until the meningococci bacteria is present in the nasal and respiratory discharge.

Clinical Manifestations:

➢ Sudden onset of fever, intense headache, nausea, and often vomiting.

➢ Sore throat, dry cough, blocked nose.

➢ Fatigue, weakness, loss of appetite, lack of sleep.

➢ Neck stiffness and frequent rash with pink macules.

➢ **Kernig's sign** may be positive (Severe stiffness of hamstring causes inability of the leg to straighten).

➢ **Brudinski's sign** may be positive (i.e. severe stiffness of the neck).

Prevention and Control: The most effective way to prevent meningitis is

• Vaccination against the disease.

• Keep distance from infected people.

• Boost your immune system.

• Avoid sharing items such as drinking glasses, water bottles, straws, silverware, toothbrushes, lipsticks, and cigarettes.

Ebola

Introduction: Ebola, also known as Ebola virus disease (EVD) and Ebola hemorrhagic fever (EHF) is a rare and deadly disease caused by infection with an Ebola virus.

Epidemiology: In 1976, Congo reported the first Ebola cases. Central and Western Africa experience frequent outbreaks of this disease. The average case fatality is around 50%. In 2014, In India, Kerala faced a risk of Ebola virus transmission from African visitors.

Transmission: Ebola is transmitted to the human population through close contact with the blood secretions, organs, or other bodily fluids of infected animals such as chimpanzees, gorillas, fruit bats, monkeys, etc. Ebola then spreads through human-to-human transmission via direct contact through broken skin or mucous membranes with bodily fluids, infected bedding, and clothing of infected people. Health care personnel treating Ebola patients are at risk.

Table 4.13 General characteristic features of Ebola

Ebola	
Infectious agent	**Ebola virus**
Reservoir	Certain infected animals or their carcasses are the natural reservoirs.
Incubation period	Around 2 to 21 days
Period of communicability	People remain infectious as long as their blood contains the virus.
Susceptibility	➤ Health Care workers who handle the blood and blood fluids of infected patients during the treatment. ➤ Persons having close contact with the blood and secretions of infected animals. ➤ Persons having contact with deceased Ebola patients.

Diagnosis: Antibody capture Enzyme-Linked Immuno Sorbent Assay (Elisa), cell cultures, RT -PCR, antigen capture detection test.

Clinical manifestations

➤ The first symptoms are sudden onset of fever, fatigue, muscle pain, severe headache, and sore throat.

➤ This is followed by vomiting, diarrhea, abdominal (stomach) pain, rash, symptoms of impaired kidney and liver functions, and in some cases both internal and external bleeding.

➤ Patients may rapidly progress to multi-organ failure, and shock.

Ebola

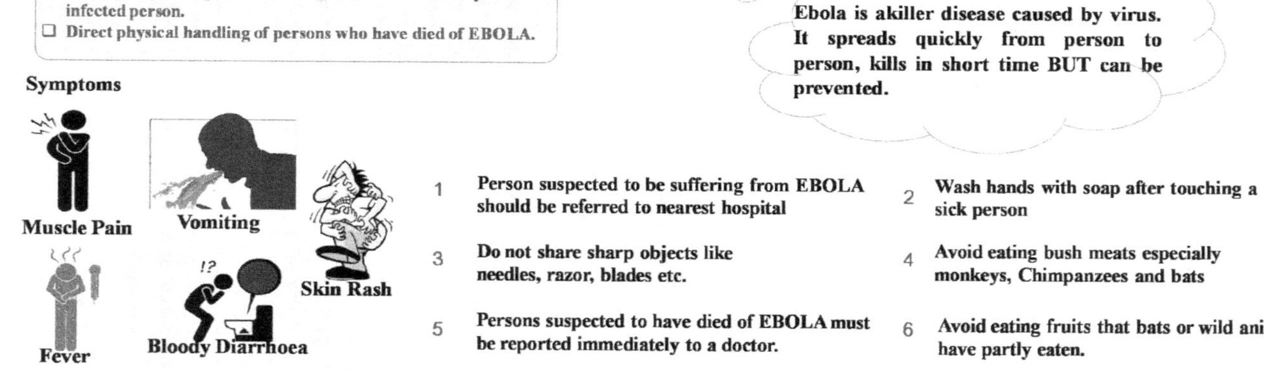

Figure 4.12 Transmission, symptoms, and preventive measures of Ebola

Prevention and Control: There is no cure for Ebola. No vaccine is available to prevent it. Health care personnel in an ebola-affected area are at high risk. These people and the close contacts of infected patients must take the following measures:

➢ Wash hands as needed, and wear protective clothing.

➢ Dispose of needles and syringes and related medical waste safely.

➢ Isolate the patient.

➢ Use safe burial practices.

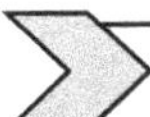 ## 4.5   Intestinal Infections

Poliomyelitis

Introduction: Polio, also known as poliomyelitis, is a disabling and life-threatening disease caused by the poliovirus. The virus transmits from person to person and can infect the spinal cord, resulting in paralysis (inability to move bodily parts).

Epidemiology: Polio was once one of the most feared diseases paralyzing hundreds of thousands of children each year. However, soon after the introduction of effective vaccines, it was brought under control. India received World Health Organization polio-free certification on March 27, 2014.

Table 4.14 General characteristic features of Poliomyelitis

Poliomyelitis	
Infectious agent	**Polio viruses (type I, II and III)**
Reservoir	humans, especially children
Incubation period	7-14 days
Susceptibility and resistance	Susceptibility is common in children but paralysis rarely occurs. Infection confers permanent immunity.
Period of communicability	Not precisely known, but transmission is possible as long as the virus is excreted.

Transmission: Polio is transmitted person-to-person principally through the fecal-oral route. Infected fingers, food, fomites, fluid (infected water), and flies transmit the disease.

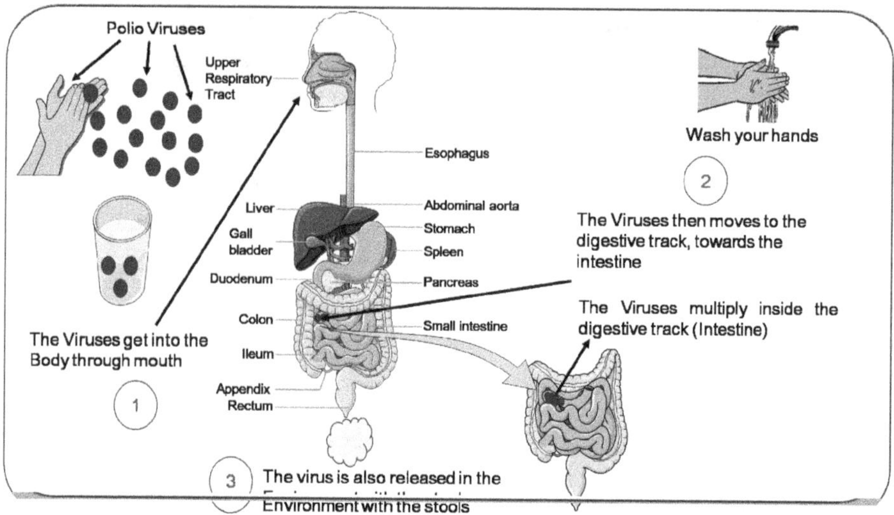

Figure 4.13 Transmission of Poliomyelitis Virus

Clinical manifestations

➤ 90% of the time, asymptomatic or non-specific fever is present. Other symptoms include sore throat, back and neck stiffness, headache, and vomiting.

➤ If the condition worsens, severe muscle pain, stiff neck and back, and flaccid paralysis may occur.

➤ Paralysis is asymptomatic and occurs within three to four days of illness.

➤ The legs are the more affected part of the body. Life Paralysis of respiratory and swallowing muscles is life-threatening

Control and Prevention

➤ Safe disposal of human excreta (feces).

➤ Educate people about early vaccination and periodic vaccination through the pulse polio program

➤ Educate people about the advantage of immunization in early childhood.

➤ Pharmacists can play important role in disease prevention by campaigning for and delivering vaccines through the pulse polio program.

Infectious Hepatitis (Viral Hepatitis-A)

Introduction: Hepatitis is an acute viral infection of liver cells that causes fever, malaise, anorexia, nausea, and abdominal pain followed by jaundice. Jaundice affects 8% of infected people. Five viruses cause viral hepatitis: Hepatitis A, B, C, D, and E. Infectious hepatitis caused by the RNA virus Hepatitis A virus (HAV), as compared to other related viruses, is more common due to its fecal-oral mode of transmission

Epidemiology: Worldwide distribution in sporadic and epidemic forms. In developing countries, adults are usually immune and epidemics of HA are uncommon. Infection is common where environmental sanitation is poor and occurs at an early age. In India, infection with HAV is most common in children below 18 years of age.

Table 4.15 General characteristic features of Viral Hepatitis

Viral hepatitis	
Infectious Agent:	***Hepatitis A virus***
Reservoir	Humans
Incubation period	10-55 days, average 28-30 days.
Susceptibility and resistance	Susceptibility is general. Immunity following infection probably lasts for life. Vaccinated persons are resistant. Attack also provides life time immunity.
Period of communicability	2 weeks before to 1 week after the onset of jaundice.

Transmission: It spreads via the fecal-oral route. Poor personal hygiene and overcrowding contribute to its spread. The pathogenic organisms are excreted in the stools of infected individuals (or, rarely, animals). This disease enters the body through the mouth. Hepatitis A is most commonly transmitted through the consumption of food and water contaminated with the feces of a Hepatitis A infected person.

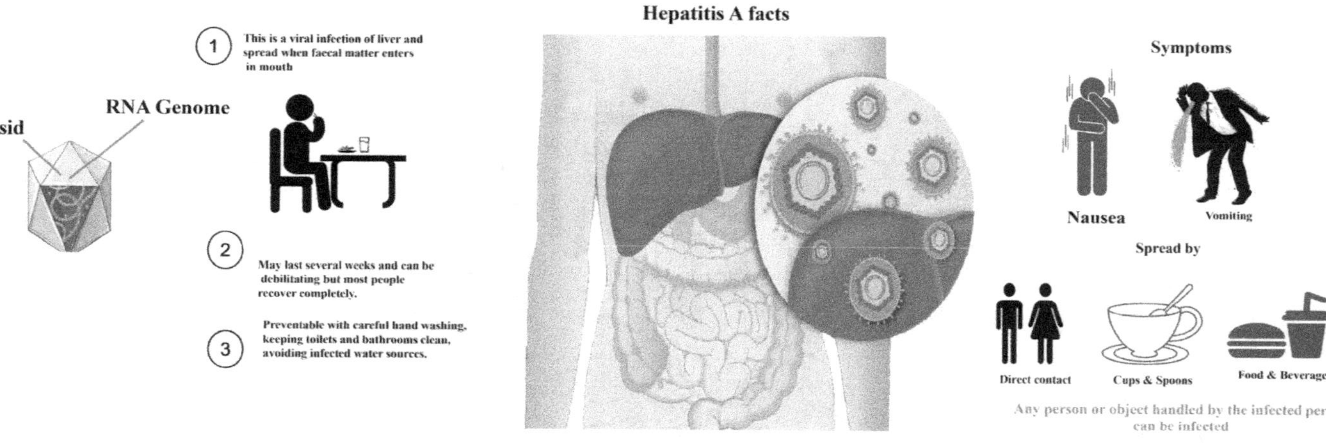

Figure 4.14 Viral hepatitis A- transmission and symptoms

Clinical manifestations: Sudden onset of fever, malaise, anorexia, nausea, stomach pain, arthralgia, headache, and photophobia, followed by jaundice with symptoms of dark yellow urine, yellow eyes, and nails. With time symptoms gradually reduce.

Diagnosis: Diagnosis can be made on the basis of clinical, and epidemiological observations and estimation of IgM antibodies (IgM anti-HAV) in the serum of acutely or recently ill patients.

Prevention and Control

1. Vaccination is important and now is included in National Immunization Program.
2. Hepatitis vaccine for all travelers to intermediate or highly endemic areas.
3. Protection of daycare center employees by the vaccine.
4. Public education about hand washing and sanitary disposal of feces.
5. Proper water treatment and distribution systems and sewage disposal.
6. Proper management of daycare centers to minimize the possibility of fecal-oral transmission.

Amoebiasis (Amoebic Dysentery)

Introduction: It is a parasitic infection of the colon with the amoeba *Entamoeba histolytica.* It may cause intestinal or extra-intestinal disease.

Epidemiology: Prevalence is worldwide but most common in the tropics and sub-tropics, particularly in areas with poor sanitation. Approximately, 10% of E histolytica infections cause invasive disease and it mostly occurs in young people (adults).

Transmission: Fecal-oral transmission by ingestion of food or water contaminated by feces containing the cysts. Fields irrigated with sewage or polluted water can readily transmit the disease. Acute amoebic dysentery poses a limited danger.

Table 4.16 General characteristic features of Amoebiasis

Amoebiasis	
Infectious agent:	*E. histolytica*
Reservoir	Humans
Incubation period	Variable from few days to several months or years; commonly 2-4 weeks.
Period of communicability	During the period of passing cysts of E. histolytica, may continue for years.
Susceptibility and resistance	Susceptibility is general. Susceptibility to reinfection has been demonstrated but is apparently rare.

Clinical Manifestation

➢ Acute amoebiasis begins with a prodromal episode of diarrhoea, the passage of 3 to 8 stools per day, abdominal cramps, nausea, vomiting, and fatigue.

➢ Excessive gas, rectal pain while having a bowel movement (tenesmus).

➢ With dysentery, feces are generally watery, containing mucus and blood.

➢ Amoebic rectal ulceration.

➢ Liver abscess and lung abscess in chronic and serious amoebic infections.

Diagnosis: Demonstration of Entamoeba histolytica cysts or trophozoites in the stool.

Prevention and Control

1. Adequate treatment of cases (Metronidazole or Tinidazole).
2. Provision of safe water for drinking and cooking and brushing teeth.
3. Proper disposal of human excreta (feces) and proper hand washing following defecation.
4. Cleaning and cooking of local foods (e.g. raw vegetables) to avoid eating food contaminated with feces. Avoid ice cubes or fountain drinks.
5. Advising periodic examination and hygiene awareness programs for cooks, and food handlers.

Cholera

Introduction: It is a severe illness caused by enterotoxin produced by *Vibrio cholera*. If not treated properly, the infection causes severe watery diarrhoea, which can lead to dehydration and even death.

Epidemiology: Cholera has become a serious disease, killing approximately 1 lakh people each year. It is most common in children. It causes periodic outbreaks in various parts of the world.

Table 4.17 General characteristic features of Cholera

Cholera	
Infectious agent:	*Vibrio cholera*
Reservoir	Humans
Incubation period	From a few hours to 5 days, usually 2-3 days.
Period of communicability	For the duration of the stool positive stage, usually only a few days after recovery. Antibiotics shorten the period of communicability.
Susceptibility and resistance	Variable. Gastric achlorhydria increases the risk of illness. Breastfed infants are protected.

Transmission: Transmitted by the ingestion of food or drink contaminated with the feces or vomitus of an infected individual, either directly or indirectly. Raw or undercooked fish captured in sewage-polluted seas, municipal water sources, ice made from municipal water, street foods, and vegetables are grown in sewage-polluted water is also risky.

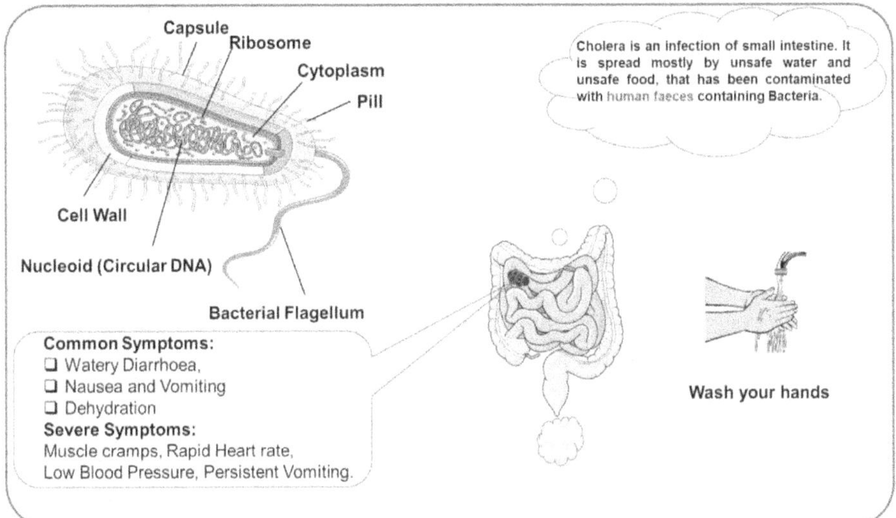

Figure 4.15 Transmission of Cholera

Clinical Manifestation

- ➢ Sudden onset of painless watery diarrhea.
- ➢ In severe cases, several liters of liquid may be lost in a few hours leading to shock.
- ➢ Dry mucous membranes, including the inside of the mouth, throat, nose, and cyelids, and muscle cramps.
- ➢ Cyanosis, sunken eyes and cheeks, low skin turgor, and a weak pulse are all symptoms of severe illness.
- ➢ Fall in blood pressure, rapid heart rate and diminished urine output.
- ➢ If not treated, it may result in death due to circulatory failure in severely dehydrated patients.

Prevention and control

- ➢ Avoid consuming unpeeled fruits and vegetables, unpasteurized milk, and milk products.
- ➢ Avoid raw or undercooked meat.
- ➢ Cook food properly, and wash hands properly.
- ➢ Drink and use safe water to brush teeth.

➤ Chemoprophylaxis with tetracycline.

➤ Vaccines: Dukoral, Sanchol, Vaxchora

Acute Diarrheal Diseases

Introduction: *Diarrhea* is a clinical syndrome characterized by the passage of unusually loose or watery bowel movements on a regular basis, usually three or more in a 24-hour period, and is sometimes accompanied by vomiting, fever, abdominal pain or cramps, fecal urgency, tenesmus (the feeling that you need to pass stools, even though your bowels are already empty), or the passage of bloody or mucoid stools. **Acute watery diarrhea** starts suddenly and lasts for less than 14 days.

Epidemiology: The disease is common in developing countries, where an estimated 4 million children under the age of five die each year. Dehydration, or the loss of fluid and electrolytes, causes nearly 80% of diarrhea-related deaths in the first two years of life. Malnutrition and dysentery are the other two major causes.

Table 4.18 General characteristic features of Acute Diarrheal disease

ACUTE DIARRHEAL DISEASES	
Infectious agent	*Rotavirus, E. coli, Shigella, Campylobacter jejuni, Cryptosporidium*
Reservoir	Drinking water contaminated with fecal bacteria
Incubation period	12-48 hours
Period of communicability	Few hours to 5 days in bacterial infection
Susceptibility and resistance	Universal, almost everyone is susceptible.

Important pathogens: Diarrhoea can result from viral, bacterial, or parasitic infections. Several of these pathogens are important causes of acute diarrhoea in all developing countries:

*Rotavirus***:** In children, rotavirus is the most prevalent cause of severe, recurring, life-threatening diarrhoea.

Vibrio cholerae releases cholera toxin which causes a profuse secretion of water and electrolytes in the small bowel followed by severe diarrhoea leading to dehydration and collapse within a few hours.

Enterotoxigenic *Escherichia coli* (ETEC) produces two types of toxins: heat-labile (LT) and heat-stable (ST) ETECs. The LT toxin is closely related to cholera toxin and is responsible for causing acute watery diarrhea.

Shigella, the most common cause of dysentery has four serotypes.

S. dysenteries type 1 causes the most severe illness because it produces Shiga toxin which causes tissue destruction and watery diarrhea.

Campylobacter jejune is the most common cause of acute diarrhea and dysentery in infants. Fever is frequently accompanied by a mild sickness that lasts two to five days.

Cryptosporidium is a common cause of recurrent diarrhea and wasting that affects infants, and immune-compromised patients.

Salmonella is one of the causes of acute watery diarrhea in areas where commercially processed foods are extensively consumed.

Transmission: Acute diarrheal infections are normally communicated by unclean hands or consumption of contaminated foods and drinks, but they can also be transmitted through aerosol dispersed by contaminated vomitus droplets. In institutions and child care centers, outbreaks are possible.

Clinical manifestation: Acute diarrheal illnesses are characterized by the abrupt onset of frequent loose or watery stools, which are frequently accompanied by vomiting and fever. The disease is usually minor and recovers on its own. In severe cases, dehydration, undernutrition, and even death due to shock may develop.

Prevention and Control: The following measures are suggested for prevention and control-

➤ Fluid and electrolyte replacement.

➤ Maintain good personal hygiene and food hygiene. Avoid drinks with ice of unknown origin. Purchase fresh food from hygienic and reliable sources.

➤ If experiencing vomiting or diarrhea, avoid going to work or school and seek medical attention. Immediate hospitalization in case of emergency.

➤ Maintain good sanitation and drainage systems. Safe disposal of young children's stools. Clean and disinfect infected people's toilets.

➤ Breastfeeding is best for babies.

Typhoid

Introduction: Typhoid fever is also called enteric fever. It is a prospectively, multisystemic illness that has been a public health problem, especially in the developing world. It is caused by *Salmonella typhi* and *Salmonella paratyphi.*

Epidemiology: Typhoid fever is most prevalent in an impoverished populations of developing countries. It causes approximately 22 million cases and 600,000 deaths every year worldwide. In endemic areas preschool and school-aged children (5-19 years of age) are most affected. 2.5% of patients become permanent carriers.

Table 4.19 General characteristic features of Typhoid

Typhoid	
Infectious agent:	*Salmonella typhi & S. paratyphi A and B*
Reservoir	Humans
Incubation period	10-14 days, bat can range from 4-21 days
Period of communicability	As long as the bacilli appear in excreta. 1-2 weeks after the temperature comes down.
Susceptibility and resistance	Susceptibility is increased in persons with gastric achlorhydria or those who are HIV positive.

Transmission: Typhoid fever and paratyphoid fever are often transmitted through the consumption of drinking water or food contaminated with the feces of individuals infected with typhoid fever or paratyphoid fever, or of individuals who are chronic carriers of the typhoid bacteria.

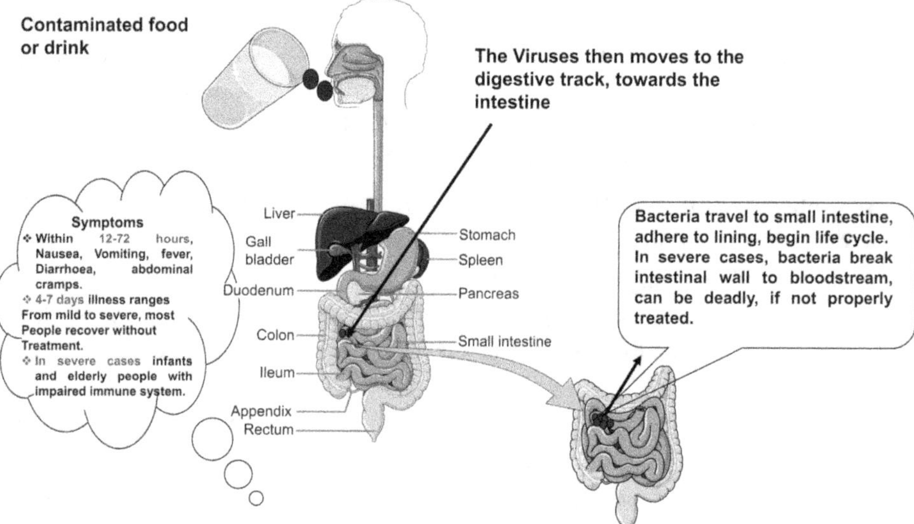

Figure 4.16 Transmission of Typhoid

Clinical manifestations

> **First week-** Mild illness characterized by **fever rising stepwise (ladder type)**, anorexia, lethargy, malaise, and general aches. Dull and continuous frontal headache is prominent. Nose bleeding, vague abdominal pain, and constipation in 10% of patients.

> **Second week- Sustained temperature** (fever). Severe illness with weakness, mental dullness or delirium, abdominal discomfort and distension. Diarrhea is more common than first week and feces may contain blood.

➢ **Third week-** Patient continues to be febrile and increasingly exhausted. If no complications occur, the patient begins to improve and the temperature decreases gradually.

➢ **Other symptoms**: Rose spots- Small pallor, blanching, slightly raised macules usually seen on the chest and abdomen in the first week in 25% of white people.

Diagnosis: Widal Test, blood, feces or urine culture.

Prevention and control:

1. Vaccination against typhoid fever.
2. Treatment of patients and carriers
3. Avoid raw, unpeeled fruits and vegetables and undercooked food.
4. Drinking only bottled/ boiled water
5. Education on hand washing, particularly food handlers, patients and childcare givers.
6. Safe handling of food.
7. Sanitary disposal of feces, and control of flies.

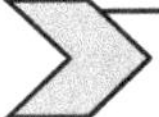 **4.6   Worm Infestations**

These illnesses spread through human contact with feces-contaminated soil.

Ascariasis

The largest nematode parasitic on the human gut is *Ascaris lumbricoides*. (roundworm) This intestinal worm lives in the small intestine. Children are more susceptible to them than adults. A single host can house anywhere from 500 to 5000 mature worms.

Epidemiology: It is the most common parasite of humans where sanitation is poor. School children (5-10 years of age) are most affected. Worldwide, 1.3 billion people are affected out of these only 120-220 million cases are symptomatic. The disease is most common in tropical and subtropical climates, as well as in areas with poor sanitation. Approximately, 10,000 people (mainly children) each year die of severe ascariasis.

Transmission: The infection is spread mostly through the intake of *A. lumbricoides* eggs in contaminated water or food (especially raw vegetables and fruits). Children may contract the parasite from their hands while playing in polluted soil. Inhalation of polluted dust is also a possibility.

Table 4.20 General characteristic features of Ascariasis

ASCARIASIS	
Infectious agent	*Ascaris lumbricoides*
Reservoir	Humans; ascaris eggs in the soil
Incubation period	4-8weeks.
Period of communicability	As long as mature fertilized female worms live in the intestine. The usual life span of the adult worm is 12 months.
Susceptibility	All are susceptible

Clinical manifestations

➢ The majority of infections go unnoticed until a huge worm is passed in the feces and, in rare cases, from the mouth and nose.

➢ Itching, wheezing, and dyspnea may be caused by migrant larvae, as well as fever and a cough with bloody sputum.

➢ Intestinal or duct (biliary, pancreatic) obstruction can cause abdominal pain.

➢ Bowel blockage from knotted/intertwined worms is a serious problem.

➢ The adult worms pass through the anus during defecation.

Prevention and Control

➢ Case management with available drugs Albendazole, Mebendazole, Piperazine, or Levamisole.

➢ Proper feces disposal.

➢ Prevent soil contamination in children's play areas.

➢ Encourage good personal hygiene.

➢ Periodic deworming for children.

Ancyclostomiasis

Introduction: Hookworms are blood-feeding parasitic nematodes that live in a human host's small intestine.

➢ *Ancylostoma duodenale* (old hookworm) and *Necator americanus* (the New World hookworm) are two hookworm species that often infect people.

➢ *Ancylostoma duodenale* is a common human hookworm that causes ancylostomiasis and manifests as non-deficiency anaemia and hypoalbuminemia. *Necator americanus* causes necatoriasis.

Epidemiology: Today, both hookworm species infect an estimated 576-740 million people, with 80 million of them being severely affected. Infection is most prevalent among the world's poorest people. Hookworm infection can hinder growth, physical fitness, and intellectual and cognitive development.

Table 4.21 General characteristic features of Ancyclostomiasis

Ancyclostomiasis (Hook worm)	
Infectious agent	*Ancylostoma duodenale* and *Necator americanus*
Reservoir	Humans; eggs in the soil
Incubation period	Few weeks to months
Period of communicability	In the absence of treatment, infected persons can contaminate the soil for years.
Susceptibility	Susceptibility is universal, No evidence that immunity develops with infection.

Transmission: Hookworms (Necator and Ancylostoma) are spread by walking barefoot on infested soil or by swimming in contaminated water. Human habits like walking without shoes, open-air defecation, and using untreated sewage water for irrigation promote the spread of diseases. Larvae enter the body by penetrating the skin. Skin penetration by third-stage larva causes intensely pruritic dermatitis called ground itch. Hookworm infection is more common on sandy soils with silt, which explains the high prevalence of hookworm infection in coastal areas.

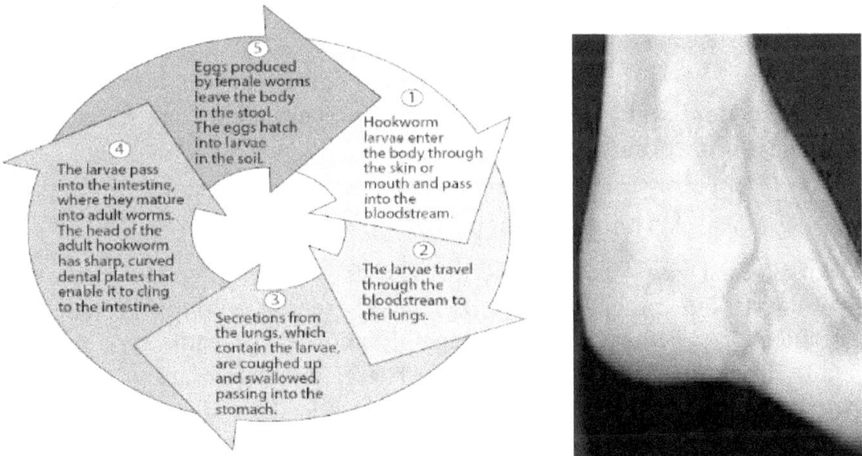

Figure 4.17 Hook worm infestation showing cutaneous larva migrants

Clinical manifestations

- ➤ **Ground itch** occurs when the L3 larva penetrates the skin. It is localized to the site of the Hookworm entry. Itching, edema, and rash are symptoms. It's likely caused by allergic components of larvae.

- ➤ **Cutaneous larva migrants** (creeping eruptions) is caused by the migration of hookworm larva in the epidermis. Lesions are seen in and around the feet, particularly between the toes.

- ➤ During the pulmonary stage, it is associated with low-grade fever, mild cough dizziness and hemolysis, sneezing, bronchitis, and pneumonia (Loeffler syndrome).

- ➤ With oral infection, nausea, vomiting, pharyngeal irritation, cough, and dyspnea might occur (Wakana syndrome).

- ➤ Once worms reach the small intestine, nonspecific abdominal symptoms might occur, such as abdominal pain and distension, nausea, vomiting, and hemorrhagic diarrhea

- ➤ Chronic hookworm disease is characterized by blood loss and Iron-deficiency anemia and is associated with fatigue, tachycardia, and dyspnea on exertion.

- ➤ In children, there may also be adverse effects on physical growth and intellectual growth.

Prevention and Control

1. Using sanitary toilet facilities.

2. Preventing the skin from directly contacting the soil (for example, by wearing shoes and using a cover or other barrier when seated on the ground)

3. Treating dogs and cats for hookworm to prevent them from spreading animal hookworms to people.

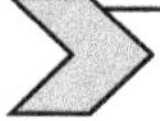

4.7   Arthropod-Borne Infections

Vector-Borne Disease is a disease that results from an infection transmitted to humans and other animals by blood-feeding anthropods such as mosquitoes, black flies, ticks, and bugs. Examples of vector-borne diseases include Dengue fever, malaria, etc. These infections are also termed **arboviral infections.** Arboviruses are viruses that are transmitted by hematophagous (feeding on blood) arthropods like mosquitoes to susceptible vertebrate hosts like a man.

Dengue

Introduction: Dengue fever also known as break bone fever is an infectious disease caused by the dengue virus. Dengue fever virus (DENV) is an RNA virus. The virus is transmitted by arthropods (mosquitoes or ticks). Dengue is transmitted by several species of mosquito within the genus Aedes, principally *A.aegypti.*

Epidemiology: Dengue occurs in >100 countries worldwide. All 4 serotypes are prevalent, Viruses are prevalent all over India except Himalayan region & Kashmir. Severe epidemics have been observed recently in north India.

In India, the reason behind the upsurge of the infection is due to uncontrolled urbanisation and population growth that have led to substandard housing, inadequate water, sewer and waste management. Ineffective mosquito control in endemic regions has further aggravated the problem.

Table 4.22 General characteristic features of Dengue

Dengue fever	
Infectious agent:	Single-stranded RNA viruses of the genus **Flavivirus** 4 serotypes of virus: Den 1-4 are prevalent.
Reservoir	Humans
Vector	**Aedes aegypti** *and* **A. albopictus**
Incubation period-	**2-7 days**
Period of communicability	Infected person becomes infective to mosquitoes 6-12hour before onset of disease and remains so up to 3-5 days.
Susceptibility and resistance	Children under 15 years of age are more susceptible

Transmission

Aedes mosquitoes are the primary carriers of transmission. Because of the approximately 7-day viral load in humans, blood-borne transmission is possible through exposure to infected blood, organs, or other tissues, also from infected mother to baby. Dengue viruses may also be transmitted through breast milk. Infection with one the four strains of dengue virus usually produces immunity to that strain but does not provide protection against other strains.

Clinical Manifestations: Signs and symptoms include-

➢ Sudden-onset of fever; 103-104^{0}F. Fever may be biphasic, initially it subsides in 2-7 days, but the other symptoms persist.

➢ Severe muscle and joint aches (myalgia and arthralgia). For this reason, it is called "break-bone fever".

➢ Characteristic skin rash that is similar to measles and facial flush. The rash develops on the feet or legs three to four days after the beginning of fever.

➢ Hemorrhagic manifestations, leukopenia and hepatomegaly

➢ Retro-orbital pain is associated with a severe headache.

Laboratory diagnosis

➢ Isolation of virus from serum.

➢ Demonstration of dengue virus antigen in serum.

➢ Detection of dengue virus genome by PCR.

Prevention and Control: The prevention of dengue requires the control or eradication of the mosquitoes carrying the virus. Anti-mosquito measures like prevention of mosquito breeding and avoiding mosquitoes from biting. For that following measures may be used.

➢ Elimination of breeding sites for mosquitos like draining coolers, emptying buckets, plant saucers, covering open tanks, etc.

➢ Using bed nets, especially, the patients need to be kept under mosquito netting until the second phase of fever is over and they are no longer contagious.

➢ Wear long-sleeved clothes even during the day time as "Aedes" mosquitoes usually bite during the day.

➢ Using in-house spraying and insect repellants, mosquito repellant coils, and vaporizers.

➢ Larvicide treatment is another effective way to control the vector larvae but the larvicide chosen should be long-lasting.

Dengue hemorrhagic fever (DHF) is more severe and is associated with loss of appetite, vomiting, high fever, headache, and abdominal pain. Shock and circulatory failure may occur. Untreated hemorrhagic dengue results in death in 50% of the cases. There is no specific treatment till date. Intravenous fluid and oxygen therapy are often used for patients, who experience shock during their illness.

Malaria

Malaria is a potentially life-threatening parasitic disease. It is a mosquito-borne acute infectious disease of humans and other animals caused by a parasitic protozoan of the genus plasmodium

Epidemiology: Malaria affects 40% of the world's population and is mostly found in tropical and subtropical regions of the world. Children under the age of five, pregnant women, and travelers to endemic areas are high risk groups. Malaria is endemic in India; however, transmission intensities vary across the country, with only a few states in the east, central, and northeast accounting for the majority (80 percent) of total positive cases.

Table 4.23 General characteristic features of Malaria

MALARIA	
Infectious agent/ Incubation period-	*Plasmodium falciparum*: **7-14 days** *Plasmodium virvax*: **8-14 days** *Plasmodium ovale*: **8-14 days** *Plasmodium malariae*: **7-30 days**
Reservoir	Humans
Period of communicability	Mosquitoes are infective as long as infective gametocytes are present in the blood of patients. Once infected, mosquito remains infective for life.
Susceptibility and resistance	Susceptibility is universal. Some people after repeated infections develop species and strain-specific humoral and cell-mediated immunity. Sickle cell traits are resistant to *Plasmodium falciparum*.

Transmission: Malaria is more common during the rainy season and is widespread in tropical regions that provide suitable environments for plasmodium to survive. Only Anopheles mosquitoes can transmit malaria and they must have been infected through a previous blood meal taken from an infected person. Transfusion of blood from infected persons and the use of contaminated needles and syringes are other potential modes of transmission.

Clinical manifestations: Symptoms appear between 7 and 18 days after becoming infected.

➤ The first symptoms of malaria are non-specific e.g. headache, fatigue, abdominal discomfort, and muscle and joint pain.
➤ Usually followed by shaking chills, fever, and profuse sweating, anorexia, nausea, vomiting.
➤ Hemolytic anemia: the parasite infects and destroys red blood cells resulting in fatigue due to anemia. jaundice. splenomegaly.
➤ Dark pigmented urine (black water fever), loose stools.
➤ Parasites can be carried by the blood to the brain (cerebral malaria, convulsions, and loss of consciousness) and to other vital organs.
➤ Malaria in pregnancy poses a substantial risk to the mother, the fetus, and the newborn infant. Pregnant women are less capable of coping with and clearing malaria infections, adversely affecting the unborn fetus.

Diagnosis is made based on the Clinical manifestation and epidemiological grounds and   examination of blood film for hemo parasite.

Prevention and Control

1. **Chemoprophylaxis**: for those who go to endemic areas but not for those who live in the endemic area (travelers and newcomers); for under-five children and pregnant mothers who have not enough immunity.

2. **Chemotherapy of cases**: Antimalarial drugs include: Chloroquine, Atovaquone, Proguanil, Artemether, Lumefantrine, Mefloquine, Quinine, Doxycycline (with quinine), Clindamycin (with quinine) and Artesunate.

3. **Vector control:** Avoiding mosquito breeding sites, spraying DDT and other chemicals, and using larvicides at breeding areas.

4. **Personal protection** against mosquito bite (use of bednets wearing full sleeve cloth.

Lymphatic Filariasis

Lymphatic filariasis (LF) is considered globally a neglected tropical disease (NTD). It is a parasitic disease caused by microscopic, thread-like worms. This disease belongs to the group of diseases called helminthiasis. The causative worms are spread by blood-feeding black flies and mosquitoes.

Epidemiology: Widely prevalent in tropical and subtropical areas of Africa, Asia, Pacific Region, Central and South America. India has 40% of the world's lymphatic filariasis (LF) cases. In India, About 31 million people are estimated to have microfilaria and over 23 million suffer from filaria disease manifestations. State of Bihar has highest endemicity (over 17%) followed by Kerala (15.7%) and Uttar Pradesh (14.6%). People living for a long time in tropical or sub-tropical areas where the disease is common are at the greatest risk for infection. Short-term tourists have a very low risk as many mosquito bites over several months to years are needed to get lymphatic filariasis.

Transmission: Adult worms' nest in the lymphatic vessels and disrupt the normal function of the lymphatic system. The worms can live for approximately 6–8 years and, during their lifetime, produce millions of microfilariae (immature larvae) that circulate in the blood. A mosquito is the intermediate host and carrier. Mosquitoes get infected with microfilariae by ingesting blood when biting an infected host. Microfilariae mature into infective larvae within the mosquito. When infected mosquitoes bite people, mature parasite larvae are deposited on the skin from where they can enter the body. The larvae then migrate to the lymphatic vessels where they develop into adult worms, thus continuing a cycle of transmission. Lymphatic filariasis is transmitted by different types of mosquitoes for example: the *Culex, Anopheles,* and *Aedes.*

Table 4.24 General characteristic features of Filariasis

FILARIASIS	
Infectious agent	***Wucheriria bancrofti*** /vectors are culex, Anopheles and Aedesspecies ***Brugia malayi*** / vector is mansonia species) ***Brugia timori*** / vector is Anopheles
Reservoir	Humans are definitive hosts.
Incubation period	One month
Period of communicability	Humans may infect mosquitoes when microfilariae are present in the peripheral blood. Microfilaremia may persists for 5-10 years or longer. The mosquito becomes infective about 12-14 days after an infective blood meal.
Susceptibility and resistance	Universal, susceptibility to infection is probable.

Clinical Manifestation: The presence of worms in the lymph vessels gives rise to a foreign-body reaction. After the death of the worm, more proteins are released; the reaction then is even more severe. Three phases may be distinguished.

Acute phase: Starts within a few months after infection, microfilariae are not seen in the peripheral blood film because the worms are not yet mature. The acute phase is mainly due to a hypersensitivity reaction.

Subacute phase: This occurs after about one year following acute phases. In this phase worms have matured and microfilariae are present in the peripheral blood.

Chronic phase: After many years of repeated attacks, lymph glands and lymph vessels become obstructed; as a result lymph edema develops but microfilariae arenot seen in the blood.

➤ Most infected people are asymptomatic but they can infect others. A small percentage of persons will develop **lymphedema**.

➤ Lymphatic filariasis impairs the lymphatic system and can lead to the abnormal enlargement of body parts, causing pain, severe disability and social stigma.

➤ This mostly affects the legs, but can also occur in the arms, breasts, and genitalia. Most people develop these symptoms years after being infected. Men can develop **hydrocele** or swelling of the scrotum.

➤ These people will have more bacterial infections in the skin and lymphatic system. This causes hardening and thickening of the skin, which is called **elephantiasis**.

➢ Filarial infection can also cause tropical pulmonary eosinophilia syndrome (Symptoms of tropical pulmonary eosinophilia syndrome include cough, shortness of breath, and wheezing).

➢ Kidney damage.

Diagnosis: A blood smear examination can easily identify the microfilaria.
Prevention and Control: World Health Organization recommends the following measures

Interruption of disease transmission is done by mass drug administration (MDA) (Mass deworming). A single dose of albendazole every year, along with either ivermectin or diethylcarbamazine citrate is administered to entire groups of individuals at risk.

Treatment: DEC is given annually for some years. Surgical treatment of hydrocele is advised.

Chikungunya

Introduction: Chikungunya is a mosquito-borne disease caused by the chikungunya virus. Chikungunya virus is most often spread to people by *Aedes aegypti* and *Aedes albopictus* mosquitoes. These are the same mosquitoes that transmit the dengue virus.

Epidemiology: Chikungunya fever is endemic in Africa, Southeast Asia, the Indian subcontinent, the Pacific region, and most probably in the sub-tropical regions of the Americas. Chikungunya fever has caused numerous epidemics in Africa and Asia. Chikungunya virus has now spread to more than 100 countries and is listed on the WHO **Blueprint priority pathogens.**

Table 4.25 General characteristic features of Chikungunya

Chikungunya	
Infectious agent	**Chikungunya virus single-stranded RNA virus**
Reservoir	Humans
Incubation period	The incubation period is usually 3-7 days (range 1-12 days).
Period of communicability	From the date of onset of symptoms to 12 days after the onset of symptoms. As CHIKV infections cause high levels of viral load, that lasts for 4 – 6 days but can persist for up to 12 days after the onset of illness.
Susceptibility and resistance	It is expected that all are susceptible. It appears that infection with CHIKV results in long-term immunity to future infection.

Transmission: Chikungunya is a mosquito-borne disease. Humans are the preferred source of blood meals for female *Aedes aegypti* mosquitoes, which are daytime biting mosquitoes. Mosquitoes become infected when they feed on a person already infected with the virus. Infected mosquitoes can then spread the virus to other people through bites.

Clinical Manifestations: Primary clinical symptoms are:

➢ Sudden onset of high fever, often reaching 102°-105°F, with shaking chills that last 2-3 days.

➢ Sore throat, abdominal pain, constipation, headache, and retro-orbital pain.

➢ Arthritis, polyarthralgia, myalgia, arthralgia- Persistent severe arthralgia could lead to long-term disability.

➢ Headache, nausea/vomiting.

➢ Maculopapular skin rash and conjunctivitis, hearing loss.

➢ Some serious clinical signs and symptoms are hepatitis, acute renal disease, cranial nerve palsies, etc.

Prevention of Chikungunya

There is neither a chikungunya virus vaccine nor drugs available to cure the infection. Prevention is the only option. That can be done by:

✓ Eliminating mosquito breeding sites is a key prevention measure.

✓ To prevent mosquito bites use mosquito repellents on skin and clothing. Use mosquito nets when sleeping.

✓ When working outdoors during the day times, wear long-sleeved shirts and long pants to avoid mosquito bites.

Control of breeding of *Aedes* mosquitos: Source reduction method

✓ Eliminate all potential vector breeding places near the domestic areas.

✓ Don't store water for more than a week. This could be done by emptying and drying the water containers once a week.

✓ Pyrethrum extract (0.1% ready-to-use emulsion) can be sprayed in rooms (not outside) to kill the adult mosquitoes hiding in the house.

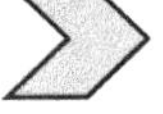

4.8   Surface Infections

Leprosy

Introduction: Leprosy (also known as Hansen's disease) is a chronic and curable infection caused by slow-growing bacteria called *Mycobacterium leprae.* It may take up to 20 years to develop signs of the infection. With early diagnosis and treatment, the disease can be cured.

The disease can affect the nerves, skin, eyes, and lining of the nose (nasal mucosa). The bacteria attack the nerves, which can become swollen under the skin. This can cause the affected areas to lose the ability to sense touch and pain, which can lead to injuries, like cuts and burns. Generally, the skin changes color, it becomes lighter/darker, often dry /flaky, with loss of feeling, or reddish due to inflammation of the skin.

Epidemiology: Leprosy was officially eradicated in India in 2005, with the national prevalence rate falling to 0.72 per 10,000 people. However, our country still has more than half of the world's new leprosy victims. The National Leprosy Eradication Program (NLEP) of India is currently one of the world's largest leprosy eradication programs.

Table 4.26 General characteristic features of Leprosy

LEPROSY (Hansen's Disease)	
Infectious agent	*Mycobacterium leprae* is an acid-fast, gram-positive bacillus.
Reservoir	Human. Wild armadillos (transmission to humans is uncertain)
Incubation period	Average 3-6 years; range, 7 months to 20 years
Period of communicability	Mildly communicable as long as solid viable bacilli are demonstrable
Susceptibility and resistance	Children are more susceptible than adults.

Transmission: A prolonged, close contact with someone with untreated leprosy is required to catch the disease. The transmission is thought to be via nasal discharges to the skin and respiratory tract of close contacts. The skin-based transmission is also possible. Open cuts or wounds on elbows, knees, and feet that are exposed to leprosy bacteria can lead to infection.

Clinical manifestations: The onset of Leprosy is usually gradual. Leprosy primarily affects skin and peripheral nerves. It also affects the eyes and mucosal lining of the nose. The common indications are:

➢ Discolored patches of skin, usually flat, that may be numb and look faded (lighter than the skin around), thick, stiff or dry skin with lesions.

➢ Disfiguration of face, painless swelling or lumps on the face or earlobes disfiguring skin sores and growths (nodules) on the skin.

➢ Painless ulcers on the soles of feet.

➢ Loss of eyebrows or eyelashes, permanent damage to nose that can cause nose bleed and stuffy nose.

➢ Erectile dysfunction and infertility in males.

Symptoms caused by damage to the nerves are:

➢ Enlarged nerves, numbness of affected areas of the skin,

➢ Muscle weakness that leads to claw-like hands or paralysis.

➢ Eye problems may lead to blindness.

Lepra reactions are defined as episodes of acute inflammation in pre-existing lesions of leprosy. These reactions are characterized by fever and the appearance of crops of painful red papules or nodules called erythema nodosum.

Prevention and Control

➢ **Early detection** of the disease is important, since physical and neurological damage may be irreversible. Patients with leprosy should be isolated during the acute stage.

➢ **Medications:** The treatment may be initiated as prescribed by the doctor. With drugs like dapsone, clofazimine, rifampicin, etc. for a period of 2 years.

➢ **Secondary prevention**: contact tracing, early diagnosis, initiation of early treatment of infection, and chemoprophylaxis to healthy household contacts.

➢ **Vaccination:** BCG vaccination is one of the prophylactic measures for leprosy.

➢ **Health education**: In endemic areas, people should be educated to avoid living and working in overcrowded areas. They should be asked to avoid sharing clothes and personal items and maintain personal hygiene.

➢ Teach safety measures to prevent burns, ulcers, injuries, etc

➢ Teach each patient to properly dispose of nasal and lesion discharges.

Tetanus

Introduction: Tetanus is also known as lockjaw. It is an acute infectious disease caused by spores of the bacterium *Clostridium tetani*. The spores are found everywhere in the environment, particularly in soil, ash, faces of animals and humans, and on the surfaces of skin and rusty tools like nails, needles, knives, etc. Being very resistant to heat and most antiseptics, the spores can survive for years.

Epidemiology: Tetanus occurs worldwide, but is most frequent in hot and wet climates where the soil has a high organic content. Tetanus cases are still present in India, however, there is a remarkable decline in incidence from 45,948 cases in 1980 to only 35 cases in the year 2019.

Table 4.27 General characteristic features of Tetanus

Tetanus	
Infectious agent	*Clostridium tetani*
Reservoir	Soil is the main reservoir
Incubation period	Around 3-21 days (average 10)
Period of communicability	Spores may remain viable for many years in the environment
Susceptibility and resistance	Newborn babies, pregnant women, and people aged above 65-year-old. Vaccination provides resistance to disease.

Transmission: Tetanus is not infectious, unlike other vaccine-preventable infections. The spores enter the body through breaks in the skin (wounds, cuts, skin punctures with needles, injections, and injuries from contaminated objects). The unclean knife, razor, or other object used to cut a newborn's umbilical cord can infect it. The disease is caused by the action of a toxin produced by the bacteria, which damages the nerves of the infected host.

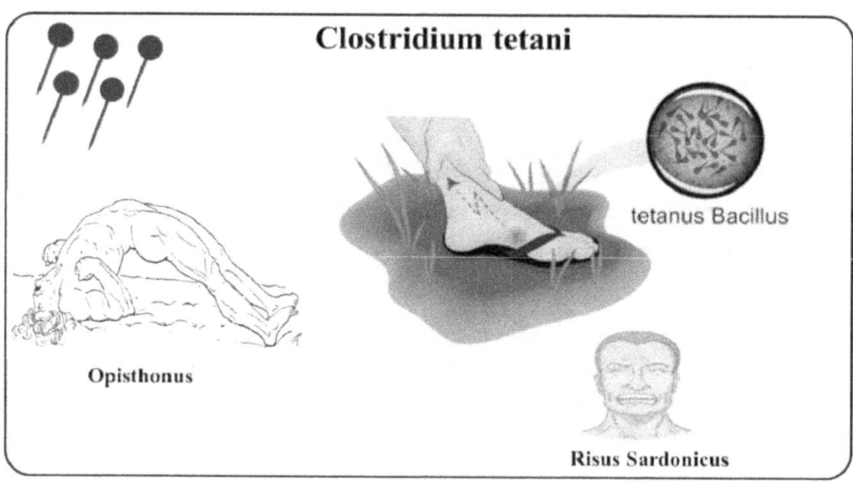

Figure 4.18 Transmission of Tetanus

Clinical manifestations: On entering any damaged tissue, the spores transform into rod-shaped bacteria and produce the neurotoxin tetanospasmin (also known as tetanus toxin). This toxin is inactive inside the bacteria, but when the bacteria die, the toxin is released and activated by proteases. Finally, it interferes with neurotransmission at the spinal synapses of inhibitory neurons.

➢ The signs and symptoms begin gradually and then progressively worsen over two weeks. These usually start at the jaw and progress downward on the body.

➢ Painful muscle spasms and stiff immovable muscles (muscle rigidity) in the jaw.

➢ Painful spasms and rigidity in neck muscles.

➢ Involuntary muscular tightness develops, and muscle contraction becomes stiff and rigid, making body movement difficult.

➢ Muscle tension around the lips, sometimes resulting in a constant grin, difficulty in swallowing, and rigid abdominal muscles.

➢ High blood pressure, fast heart rate, fever, sweating, and headache.

Prevention and Control

1. Tetanus vaccination and wound care are important in preventing tetanus infection. Routine immunization is recommended. In the event of an injury, wound, or accident, a vaccination shot should be given. Immunization is recommended during pregnancy.

2. Children should be vaccinated with different doses of DPT.

3. Use of properly autoclaved surgical instruments, and sterile and disposable syringes.

4. Wash hands often with soap and water or uses an alcohol-based hand rub.

Trachoma

Introduction: Trachoma is a chronic infectious disease of conjunctiva and cornea caused by *Chlamydia trachomatis.*

Epidemiology: Worldwide, about 21 million people have trachoma, and 2.2 million are completely blind or have severe vision impairment. In 51 nations, trachoma causes blindness. In India, it's 3.5/1000. Children are most affected in endemic areas.

Table 4.28 General characteristic features of Trachoma

Trachoma	
Infectious agent	*Chlamydia trachomatis* **serotype A, B, or C**
Reservoir	Children with active disease
Incubation period	Around 5 to 10 days
Period of communicability	2 to 3 months
Susceptibility and resistance	Most common in children of 2-5 years of age. Age above 16 and below 40 are at low risk

Transmission: Source of infection is the ocular discharges of infected persons. Trachomatis can be transmitted directly by eye, nose, and throat secretions or indirectly by fomites (inanimate objects that transport infectious organisms) such as towels, handkerchiefs, gloves, etc. Flies that have touched a patient's eyes or nose can potentially spread the disease.

Clinical manifestation: The symptoms start with mild eye itching and irritation, mucus or pus discharge, swollen eyelids, light sensitivity (photophobia), redness, and pain followed by blepharospasm (involuntary tight closure of eyelids).

The infection process starts with the appearance of very small bumps on the inner surface of the upper eyelid. Repeated infections lead to scarring of the inner side of the eyelids leading to its distortion and entropion (turning in of eyelashes). The scarred inner lining of eyelids continues to deform which causes the lashes to turn in. Such lashes rub on and scratch off the transparent outer surface of the cornea. All the symptoms are more severe in your upper lid than in your lower lid. If ignored leads to blindness.

Prevention and Control

➢ Face cleanliness: Frequent washing of the face and hands may break the cycle of infection.

➢ Environment improvement: Improvement of waste management, sanitation, and drainage system in cities and villages can reduce the number of flies that can help in the reduction of disease transmission.

➢ Regular screening and early initiation of treatment (antibiotics) in communities where trachoma is endemic.

➢ Surgery of affected people having trichiasis can prevent cases of blindness

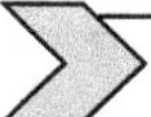

4.9   Human Immunodeficiency Virus

Introduction: Human Immunodeficiency Virus (HIV) is a retrovirus, which means it is made of RNA rather than DNA. This virus particularly infects humans. HIV attacks the immune system's most important cells, T-cells, and CD4 cells. HIV destroys the most of CD4 cells, reducing the body's ability to fight infections and illnesses, ultimately leading to the condition known as AIDS.

➢ **A – Acquired** – AIDS is not a disease inherited from one's parents. AIDS is acquired after birth.

➢ **I – Immuno** –immune system consists of all the organs and cells that fight infection and disease.

➢ **D – Deficiency** –AIDS is acquired when the immune system is "weak" or not functioning properly.

> **S – Syndrome** – A syndrome is a collection of symptoms and signs of disease.

AIDS is a syndrome, rather than a single disease because it is a complex illness with a wide range of complications and symptoms.

Acquired Immunodeficiency Syndrome is the final stage of HIV infection. People at this stage of HIV disease have badly damaged immune systems, which put them at risk for opportunistic infections.

Transmission: HIV is transmitted by three main routes: sexual contact, exposure to infected body fluids or tissues, and from mother to child.

> **Sexual transmission:** The most frequent mode of transmission of HIV is through sexual contact with an infected person.

> **Through Body fluids**: The second most frequent mode of HIV transmission is via blood and blood products. It could be through needle-sharing during intravenous drug use, transfusion of contaminated blood or blood product, or unsterilized syringes.

> **Mother-to-child (vertical transmission):** HIV can be transmitted from mother to child during pregnancy, during delivery, or through breast milk.

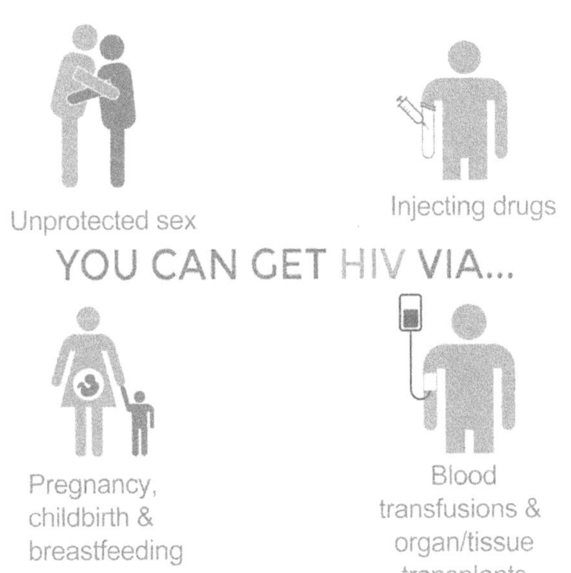

Figure 4.19 Transmission of HIV

Clinical Manifestations: There are three main stages of HIV infection: acute infection, clinical latency, and AIDS.

Acute Infection: Occurs within 2-4 weeks to 3 months after exposure to HIV. The person experiences a flu-like acute illness. The Symptoms include:

➤ Chills, recurring fever, profuse night sweats, rashes.

➤ Extreme and unexplained tiredness and muscle aches.

➤ Diarrhea that lasts for more than a week.

➤ Sores of the mouth, anus, or genitals.

➤ Prolonged swelling of the lymph glands in the armpits or neck.

This is called acute retroviral syndrome (ARS), or primary HIV infection. During this stage, there are higher levels of virus circulating in the blood, and the person can transmit the virus to others.

Clinical Latency: After the initial infection the virus becomes less active in the body, although it is still present. During this period, many people do not have any symptoms of HIV infection. This period is called the "chronic" or "latency" phase. This period can last up to 10 years sometimes longer.

AIDS: When HIV infection progresses to AIDS, many people begin to suffer from fatigue, diarrhea, nausea, vomiting, fever, chills, night sweats, and even wasting syndrome at late stages. Many of the signs and symptoms of AIDS come from opportunistic infections which occur in patients with a damaged immune system.

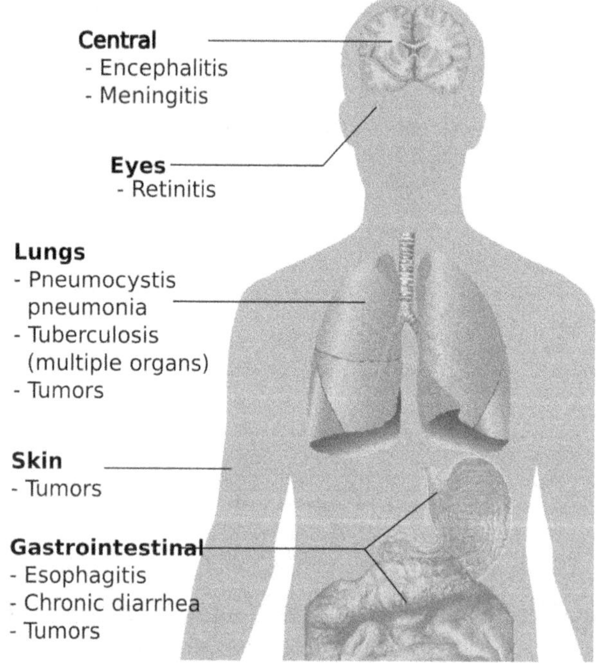

Figure 4.20 Symptoms of AIDS

Common Opportunistic Infections are:

➢ Pneumonia: Pneumocystis carinii.

➢ Oral candidiasis opportunistic infection.

➢ Toxoplasmosis of the CNS.

➢ Chronic diarrhea/wasting syndrome.

➢ Pulmonary/extra-pulmonary tuberculosis.

➢ **Cancers**: Cancers: People living with HIV or AIDS are much more likely to get certain types of cancer e.g.

   ✓ Kaposi's sarcoma – affects small blood vessels and internal organs.

   ✓ Cervical dysplasia and cancer. Researchers found out that women with HIV have higher rates of this type of cancer. Cervical carcinoma is associated with Human Papilloma Virus (HPV).

   ✓ Non-Hodgkin's lymphoma – cancerous tumor of the lymph nodes. This is usually a late manifestation of HIV infection.

Prevention and control

1. **Health education** – The healthcare workers must educate the community by giving advice.

2. **Prevention-**

1. Care should be taken to avoid accidental pricks from sharp instruments contaminated with potentially infectious materials from AIDS patients.

2. Blood and other specimens should be labeled with a special warning "AIDS Precaution".

3. Needles should not be bent after use but should be disposed into a puncture-resistant container.

4. Personal articles like razors or razor blades and toothbrushes should not be shared with other members of the family. Razor blades may be disposed of in the same manner as needles are disposed of.

5. Patients with active AIDS should be isolated.

The Four Cs in the Management of HIV/AIDS

1. Compliance: Counselling the patient to follow the treatment instructions and recommendations.

2. Counseling and educating the patient about the information related to the disease, the importance of treatment, and guidance on how to avoid its spread.

3. Contact tracing: Tracing out the contacts.

4. Condoms: Promoting the use of the condom, and giving instructions about their use.

Syphilis

Introduction: Syphilis is a disease characterized by a primary lesion followed by a secondary eruption on the skin and mucus membranes. After that, there may be a long period of latency and finally may lead to late lesions of skin, bones,viscera, CNS, and cardiovascular systems.

Epidemiology: The disease has worldwide distribution. The majority of the patients are sexually active young individuals aged 20 to 29. Urban areas have a higher prevalence than rural areas.

Table 4.29 General characteristic features of Syphilis

Infectious agent	*Treponema pallidum*
Reservoir	Humans
Incubation period	3 weeks to 20 years depending on the type
Period of communicability	Variable and indefinite, during primary and secondary stages. Up to 2 years possibly longer .
Susceptibility	Universal, approximately 30% of exposures result in infection.

Transmission: Syphilis is spread through direct contact with a chancre, also known as a syphilitic sore. Chancres (ulcers) can appear in or around the external genitalia, vagina, anus, or rectum, as well as the mouth. Syphilis can be transferred through oral, anal, or vaginal contact. In addition, pregnant mothers can transmit syphilis to their unborn children.

Clinical manifestations: Syphilis can manifest itself in a variety of ways, including no symptoms at all. It may go undetected until complications arise or a partner is diagnosed. Depending on the infecting organism, symptoms may appear days or years after exposure. Some common symptoms include:

➢ Sores on the genitals or in the oral or rectal area, rash over the trunk, hands, or feet.

➢ Painful or burning urination, lower abdominal pain.

➢ Discharge from the penis, pain during sex.

➢ Unusual or odorous vaginal discharge or bleeding.

➢ Sore, swollen lymph nodes.

➢ High fever

Prevention and Control: Syphilis does not have a vaccine. Follow these guidelines to help prevent the spread of syphilis.

➢ Treatment of cases, monthly examinations, and case management.

➢ Sexual health education, be monogamous.

➤ STD prevention among commercial sex workers.

➤ Prenatal screening and early treatment to avoid congenital syphilis.

➤ Blood screening before the transfusion.

➤ Sharing needles is another way for syphilis to spread. Educating people on the risk of sharing needles.

➤ The use of condoms can reduce your risk of contracting syphilis, but only if the condom covers the syphilis sores.

Gonorrhea

Gonorrhea is a bacterial infection spread through sexual contact and affects both men and women. The most common sites of gonorrhea include; the urethra, cervix in women, rectum, mouth, eyes, and joints.

Epidemiology: Both genders are affected, but sexually active teenagers and young adults are the most vulnerable. This is frequent in rural areas. It's especially common in low-income areas. In most developed countries, the incidence has decreased during the last two decades.

Table 4.30 General characteristic features of Gonorrhea

GONORRHEA	
Infectious agent	*Neisseria gonorrhea*
Reservoir	Humans are only being a natural reservoir
Incubation period	2 to 14 days
Period of communicability	This can persist for months in those who are not treated. Effective therapy eliminates communicability within hours.
Susceptibility	Susceptibility can affect everyone. Sexually aware people are at low risk
Resistance	Following infection, there is no immunity, and reinfection is usual.

Transmission: Having unprotected sex with someone who has the infection is the most common way to contact gonorrhea. People contract gonorrhea most commonly through vaginal, anal, or oral intercourse. The infection can also be passed on from mother to baby after childbirth.

Clinical manifestations: The genital tract is affected by gonorrhea. Men with gonorrhea may have the following signs and symptoms:

➤ Painful urination.

➤ Pain or swelling in one testicle.

➤ Pus-like secretion from the tip of the penis.

Infected women may have:

➤ Increased vaginal discharge.

➢ Painful urination.

➢ Vaginal bleeding between periods, such as after vaginal intercourse.

➢ Abdominal or pelvic pain.

Signs and symptoms of gonococcal infections at organs other than the genital tract:

➢ Rectum: Anal irritation, pus-like discharge from the rectum, bright red blood spots on toilet paper.

➢ Eyes: The infection in the eyes may cause eye pain, light sensitivity, and pus-like discharge from one or both.

➢ Throat: A painful throat and enlarged lymph nodes in the neck.

➢ Joints: While bacteria invade one or more joints (septic arthritis), the affected joints become red, swollen, and painful, especially when moving.

Prevention and Control

➢ Identification, detection, and early treatment of cases.

➢ Use of condoms during sexual contact.

➢ Avoid sexual relations with multiple partners.

➢ Health education and awareness programs about STDs.

CHAPTER 5

Introduction to Health Systems and all Ongoing National Health Programs in India

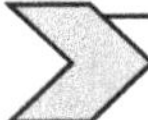 ## 5.1 Health System

LEARNING OBJECTIVES

♦ Introduction to health systems and all ongoing National Health programs in India, their objectives, functioning, outcomes, and the role of pharmacists.

> A health system is the sum total of all the organizations, institutions, and resources whose primary purpose is to improve health.

> The terms *health systems* and *healthcare systems* are often used interchangeably but there is a big difference between these. Health care systems are limited to personal healthcare services, such as curative services, whereas health systems encompass wider determinants of health, such as social and economic determinants of health

> A health system needs staff, funds, information, supplies, transport, communication, and overall guidance and direction.

> It also needs to provide services that are responsive and financially fair while treating people.

Objectives of Health System

In order to fulfil the primary purpose of improving health, a health system is required to achieve the following five fundamental objectives:

> To enhance the health status of individuals, families, and communities.

> To protect the population against what threatens its health.

> To protect people against the financial burden of any disease.

> To provide fair access to people-centered care.

> To make it feasible for people to get involved in decision-making that affects their health and health system.

Requirements for health systems: A good health system delivers quality services to all people when and where they need them. The exact structure of services differs from one country to another. But in all cases, it requires:

➤ A strong financing system that finances health care.

➤ A well-trained and adequately paid workforce that includes people that provide preventive health services, clinical services, and specialized inputs into health care.

➤ Trustworthy information that makes the basis of decision-making and framing of policies.

➤ Well-maintained facilities.

➤ Well-planned arrangements to deliver quality medicines and technology through agencies that plan, fund, and regulate health care.

Components of the Health System

The concept of a health system depends on what it is supposed to do and how it is meant to do it. This gave rise to a conceptual health system framework that can define, describe and explain the health system by elaborating its objectives, structural and organizational elements, functions, and processes.

In 2007, a framework for the health system was proposed by WHO that has the following six building blocks:

1. **Service delivery**: Good health services are those that deliver effective, safe, quality, personal, and non-personal health interventions to individuals who need them, when and where they need them with minimal waste of resources.

2. **Health workforce**: To achieve the best health outcomes the health system requires a sufficient number of competent, responsive, and productive health workforce that is evenly distributed in a geographical area.

3. **Information**: The information on health determinants, health system performance, and health status need to be reliable and must be produced, analyzed, and shared in a timely manner.

4. **Medical products, vaccines, and technology**: Access to essential medical products, vaccines, and technologies of assured quality, safety, efficacy, and cost-effectiveness is equitable and all medical products should be scientifically sound and used in a cost-effective way.

5. **Financing**: A good health financing system generates enough money for healthcare. It does it in a way that guarantees every individual has access to the services they need and also protects them from any financial hardship in case they pay for that.

6. **Leadership and governance**: Leadership and governance ensure strategic policy frameworks in a health system. They are combined with supervision, regulation, incentives, and accountability.

These six components alone do not constitute a system. It is the multiple relationships and interactions amongst these that make and strengthen a health system. Some components, such as health information and leadership and governance provide the basis for the overall policy and regulation of all the other health system blocks. Medical products, vaccines and technologies, and service delivery reflect the immediate outputs of the health system, such as the availability and distribution of care. Moreover, financing and health workforce are key components of a well-functioning health system.

All the six components are distinct, and to achieve the goals the interactions between these are essential for the health system. Therefore, all parts of the system are required to function collectively in order to be efficient.

Table 5.1 Role of pharmacist in different components of health system

S.No	Components of the health system	Role of pharmacist in the health system
1	Service delivery	➢ Pharmacists are responsible for delivering effective, safe, and quality medicines and services to achieve optimal health outcomes. ➢ They need to be competent in their field with continuous updation of knowledge.
2	Health workforce	➢ Well-performing pharmacists will provide patient-centered pharmacy service, putting the interests of patients and treating them with dignity. ➢ They are responsive to patient's needs, preferences and satisfaction in order to have reduced complaints against offered services.
3	Information	➢ Pharmacists are one of the most accessible health care professionals therefore they contribute to the development of the public health system and decrease vulnerability to public health threats by providing reliable and timely health information. ➢ It is due to their involvement in health screening, surveillance programs, checking immunization status, and detecting potential public health hazards.
4	Medical products, vaccines, and technology	➢ The availability of a wide range of newer medical products, vaccines, and technologies, demands special knowledge with regard to uses and risks. ➢ Pharmacists have a broad knowledge of all the products and technologies and are responsible for ensuring the efficacy, integrity, and security of medical products, devices, and, vaccines to safeguard a patient's health.

Table 5.1 *Contd...*

S.No	Components of the health system	Role of pharmacist in the health system
5	Financing	➢ Pharmacists ensure the provision of cost-effective health care through the rational use of medical products and modern technologies and protect vulnerable populations from financial problems related to the treatment. ➢ Pharmacists help the patients to increase their health care savings by providing cheaper alternatives or suggesting medicines that are covered by insurance and also by preventing medication-related problems
6	Leadership and governance	➢ Pharmacists take part in public health policy development; linking disease prevalence and drug utilization, ➢ Pharmacists enable the development of effective health policies, ➢ Pharmacists contribute to emergencies in terms of designing response plans and protocols, ➢ They contribute to resource mobilization through the optimization of medication use and distribution.

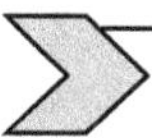

5.2   Healthcare System

Indian healthcare system: Indian healthcare system is divided into two sectors: Public and Private.

Public sector healthcare system: The public healthcare sector (run by the Government) is responsible for providing health services and treatments to all people. This sector includes super-specialty hospitals equipped with medicines and instruments, which are majorly located in tier I and tier II cities. Additionally, district and taluka-level hospitals provide healthcare services to the people. Primary healthcare centers and village hospitals provide affordable healthcare services.

Private sector healthcare: The private health sector provides healthcare services and is not owned or regulated by governments. The overall cost of healthcare services included in the private sector is higher than that in the public sector. Technological interventions are also more diverse in the private sector than in the public sector. The figure illustrates the detailed structure of the Indian healthcare system.

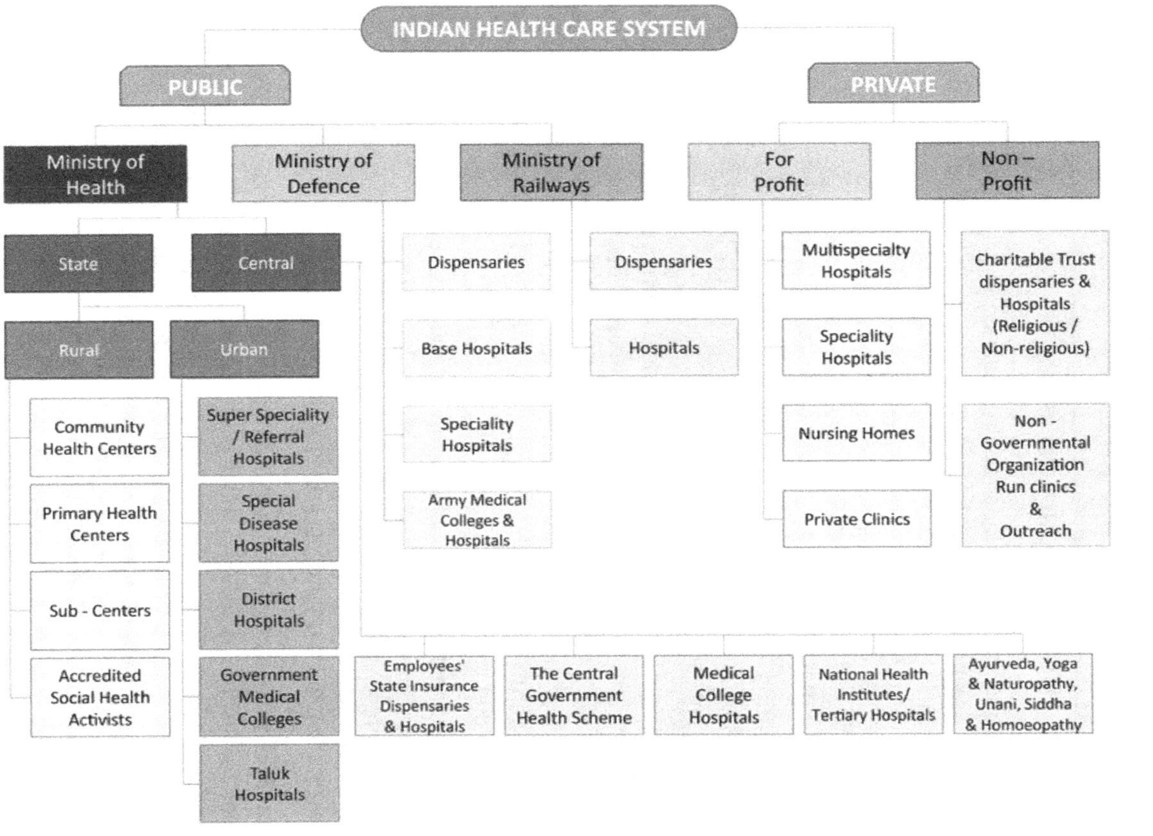

Figure 5.1 Indian Healthcare System

Non-profit hospitals: Non-profit hospitals are community hospitals and their main goal is to provide free-of-cost health services to the community. These hospitals are funded by donations and offerings made by the general public.

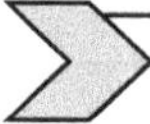 ## 5.3   National Health Programs

➢ Since its independence, India has formulated and implemented various National Health Programs that helped to improve the health status of its people.

➢ International agencies like WHO, UNICEF, etc also provide assistance in the implementation of these programs.

➢ National Programs have the following features in common:

- **Targeting one disease**: Usually, a national health program is designed to target one disease. For example, the National Malaria Program focused specifically on malaria.

- **Vertical in nature**: Every national program has a separate workforce, fund allocation and research institutes, etc, and the program is usually not integrated with the general health system. However, under the umbrella of the National Health Mission (NHM) almost all the national programs are integrated with the general national health services.

- The impact of National health programs is constantly monitored through surveillance mechanisms to check the impact on the disease burden. The focus is on both preventive and curative aspects.

IMPORTANT NATIONAL HEALTH PROGRAMS IN INDIA

National Health Programs to Control Non-Communicable Diseases: Non-communicable diseases (NCDs) are identified as one of the major challenges globally. These are the leading cause of premature death i.e., in the ages of 30 and 69 years which are preventable and avoidable. Nearly 85% of premature deaths are in low and middle-income countries.

Target 3.4 of Sustainable Development Goal 3 aims to reduce premature NCD mortality by one third by 2030. Since the adoption of the SDGs in September 2015, India has demonstrated a strong commitment and is the first country to develop specific national targets and indicators aimed at reducing the number of global premature deaths from NCDs by 25% by 2025.

Programs aimed at controlling Non - Communicable Diseases (NCDs)

1. National program for prevention and control of diabetes, cardiovascular diseases, and stroke

2. National program for control of blindness (NPCB)
3. National mental health program (NMHP)
4. National program for prevention and control of deafness
5. National program for oral health

Table 5.2 National Program for Prevention and Control of Diabetes, Cardiovascular Diseases and Stroke

<table>
<tr>
<td>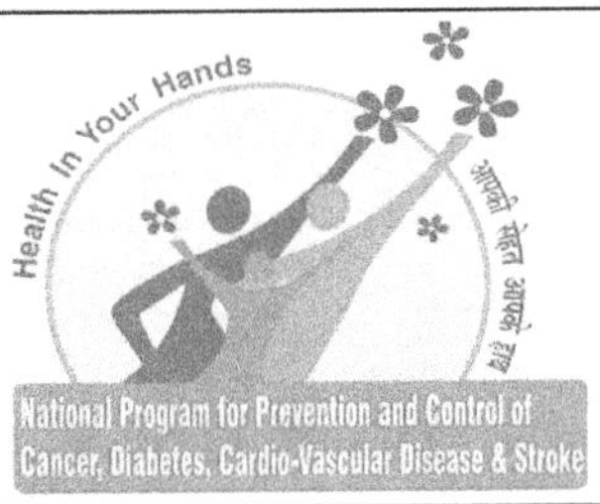</td>
<td>National Program for Prevention and Control of Cancer, Diabetes, Cardiovascular Diseases, and Stroke
Launched in 2010 by NHM</td>
</tr>
<tr>
<td colspan="2">

Goal:

Health promotion and prevention, infrastructure strengthening, early diagnosis and management, and integration with the primary health care system through NCD cells at different levels for operational efficiency.

</td>
</tr>
<tr>
<td colspan="2">

Objectives:

- To prevent and control common NCDs through behavior lifestyle changes
- To provide early diagnosis and management of common NCDs,
- To build capacity at various levels of health care for prevention, diagnosis, and treatment of common NCDs,
- To train human resources in the public health setup i.e. doctors, paramedics, and nursing staff to cope with the increasing burden of NCDs.
- To establish and develop capacity for palliative and rehabilitative care.

</td>
</tr>
<tr>
<td colspan="2">

Functioning:

- Health promotion, awareness generation, and promotion of a healthy lifestyle by focusing on increased intake of healthy foods, salt reduction, increased physical activity/regular exercise, avoidance of tobacco and alcohol, reduction of obesity, stress management, awareness about warning signs of cancer, regular health checkup, etc.
- Screening and early detection of common cancers, diabetes, and high blood pressure, through camps at different levels of health facilities and also in urban slums of large cities.
- Timely, affordable, and accurate diagnosis.
- Access to affordable treatment
- Rehabilitation

</td>
</tr>
<tr>
<td colspan="2">

Outcomes: The program is under implementation in all States/UTs. There are 667 District NCD Cells, 667 District NCD Clinics, 4406 CHC NCD Clinics, 192 Cardiac Care Units, and 217 District Day Care Units functional in the country.

</td>
</tr>
</table>

Table 5.3 National Program for Control of Blindness (NPCB)

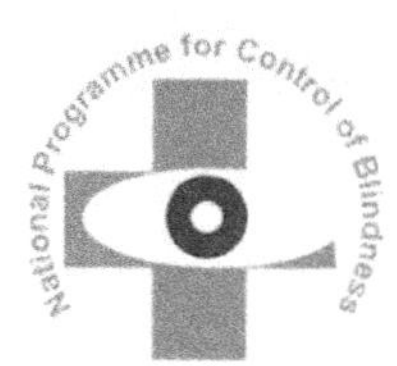

National Program for Control of Blindness (NPCB)
Vision 2020 is the right to sight
Launched in 1976

Goal:
- To reduce the prevalence of blindness from 1.49% to 0.3% by the year 2020.
- To establish infrastructure and efficiency levels in the program to be able to cater to new cases of blindness each year to prevent future backlogs.

Objectives:
- Identification and treatment of blind at primary, secondary, and tertiary levels.
- To develop comprehensive and quality eye care services.
- Strengthening and up gradation of existing ophthalmology centers.
- Strengthening of existing infrastructure facilities and human resources for providing eye care in all districts.
- To enhance community awareness of eye care.
- Increase and expand research for the prevention of blindness and visual impairment.

Functioning:
- Active screening of population above 50 years for cataracts.
- Screening of school children and women in rural areas for identification and treatment of refractive errors and other eye problems.
- By enhancing public awareness about the timely treatment of eye ailments; Emphasizing free cataract surgery through the Government health care system and through NGOs.
- Development of eye care services and improvement in quality of eye care by regular monitoring of services and training of personnel.
- Making eye care comprehensive by including eye diseases other than cataracts like diabetic retinopathy, glaucoma management, laser techniques, corneal transplantation, etc.
- Construction of dedicated eye wards and eye OTs in district hospitals in the NE States and a few other states as per need.
- Development of multipurpose district mobile ophthalmic units (MDMOU)] at the district level for patient screening & transportation.

Outcomes: 3.35 million cataract surgeries were performed, and funds were utilized for training and infrastructure development.

Table 5.4 National Mental Health Program (NMHP)

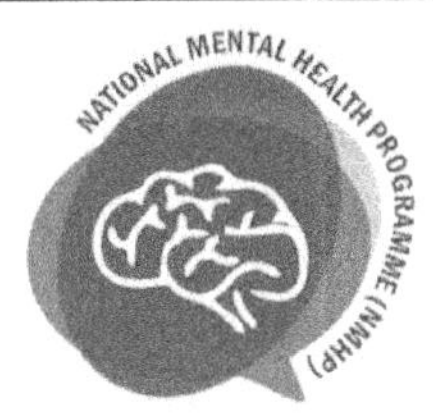

	National Mental Health Program (NMHP) Launched in 1982

Goals:
- ➤ To prevent and treat mental, and neurological disorders and to reduce distress, disability, exclusion morbidity, and premature mortality associated with mental health problems of the person.
- ➤ To strengthen the leadership in the mental health sector at the national, state, and district levels.

Objectives:
- ➤ To ensure the availability and accessibility of minimum mental health care for all.
- ➤ To encourage the application of mental health knowledge in general health care and in social development.
- ➤ To promote community participation in mental health service development and to enhance human resources in mental health subspecialties.
- ➤ To reduce the prevalence and impact of risk factors associated with mental health problems.

Functioning:
- ➤ Early diagnosis and treatment of mental illness in the community.
- ➤ Rehabilitation and promotion of positive health.
- ➤ Basic Services: Diagnosis and treatment of common mental disorders such as psychosis, depression, anxiety disorders, and epilepsy.
- ➤ Information education and communication activities for prevention, stigma removal, early detection of mental disorders, and greater participation/role of the community for primary prevention of mental disorders.

Outcomes: NMHP is implemented in all state/district levels.

Table 5.5 National program for Prevention and control of deafness

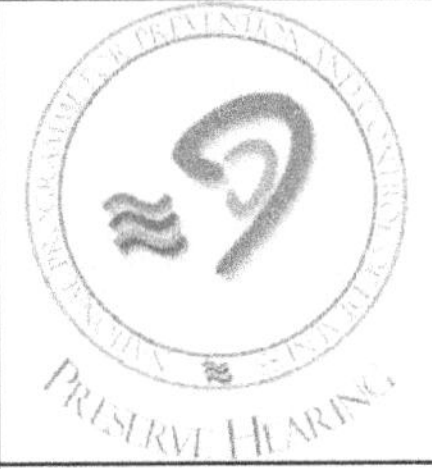

	National Program for Prevention and Control of Deafness Launched from2006 to 2008

Goals: To prevent and control major causes of hearing impairment and deafness, so as to reduce the total disease burden by 25% of the existing burden by the end of the 12th Five Year Plan.

Objectives:
- ➤ To prevent avoidable hearing loss on account of disease or injury.
- ➤ Early identification, diagnosis, and treatment of ear problems responsible for hearing loss and deafness.

Table 5.5 *Contd...*

> ➤ To medically rehabilitate persons of all age groups, suffering from deafness.
> ➤ To strengthen the existing inter-sector linkages for continuity of the rehabilitation program, for persons with deafness.
> ➤ To develop institutional capacity for ear care services by providing support for equipment, material and training personnel.

Functioning:
> ➤ Early detection and management of hearing and speech impaired cases and rehabilitation, at different levels of the health care delivery system.
> ➤ Awareness generation for early identification of hearing impaired, especially children so that timely management of such cases is possible and to remove the stigma attached to deafness.
> ➤ Development of human resources for ear care services.
> ➤ Institutional capacity of hospitals, community health centers, and primary health centers selected under the program.

Outcomes:
Availability of various services through this program (like prevention, early identification, treatment, referral, rehabilitation, etc. for hearing impairment and deafness at the primary health center/community health center/district hospitals) will decrease the magnitude of hearing impaired persons and will reduce the extent of hearing impairment.

Table 5.6 National Oral Health Program

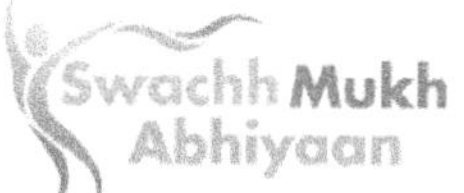	**National Oral Health Program** Launched during 2014 – 15

Goals: To prevent and control oral and craniofacial diseases, conditions, and injuries and to improve access to preventive services and dental care.

Objectives:
> ➤ To enhance the determinants of oral wellbeing.
> ➤ To reduce plaque caused by oral infections
> ➤ To incorporate oral well-being advancement and preventive administrations with a general human services framework.
> ➤ To empower promotion of Public-Private Partnerships (PPP) display for accomplishing better oral wellbeing.

Functioning:
> ➤ NHM provides support to states to set up dental units at district hospitals, to appoint dentists, dental hygienists, and dental assistants, and to have equipment including dental chairs and consumables for dental procedures.
> ➤ Increasing awareness by designing materials like posters, TV, radio spots, and training modules.
> ➤ Organizing national, and regional nodal officers training programs to enhance the program management skills, review the status of the program
> ➤ Preparing State/District level trainers by conducting nationwide regional workshops to train the paramedical health staff associated with health care delivery.

Outcomes: The awareness generation and availability of various services through this program will reduce the incidence of oral diseases.

Programs aimed at controlling Communicable Diseases

1. National vector-borne diseases control Program (NVBDCP)
2. National leprosy eradication program (NLEP): National Action Plan
3. National tuberculosis elimination program
4. National AIDS Control Program

National Vector-borne disease control program (NVBDCP): The National vector-borne Disease control program (NVBDCP) is an umbrella program for the prevention and control of malaria and other vector-borne diseases like lymphatic filariasis, kala-azar, japanese encephalitis, chikungunya and dengue with special focus on the vulnerable groups of the society namely, children, women, scheduled castes (SC) and scheduled tribes (ST). Under the program, it is ensured that the disadvantaged and marginalized sections benefit from the delivery of services so that the desired National health policy and Rural health mission goals are achieved.

Table 5.7 National Vector-borne control program (NVBDCP)

	**National Vector-borne diseases control program (NVBDCP)** (launched in 1975)

Goal: Prevention and control of vector-borne diseases namely Malaria, Dengue, Kala-azar, Filariasis, Chikungunya fever, and Japanese Encephalitis

Objectives:
- To reduce case incidence, including morbidity of Japanese encephalitis, dengue, malaria, and chikungunya by 50% by 2017.
- To achieve elimination of kala-azar and lymphatic filariasis by 2015.
- To conduct surveillance for disease outbreaks, early diagnosis, and prompt case management. Vector control through community participation and social mobilization.

Functioning:
- Diagnosis and management of vector-borne diseases to be undertaken as per NVBDCP guidelines for PHC/CHC.
- Diagnosis of malaria cases, microscopic confirmation, and treatment.
- Cases of suspected Japanese encephalitis and dengue are to be provided with symptomatic treatment, hospitalization, and case management as per the protocols.
- Complete treatment of kala-azar cases in endemic areas as per national policy.
- Complete treatment of microfilaria-positive cases with *Diethylcarbazine* and participation in Mass Drug Administration (MDA) along with management of complications.
- Formulating policies and guidelines
- Providing technical guidance to the states.
- Planning and logistics
- Monitoring and evaluation.

Table 5.7 *Contd...*

> Coordination of activities through states/UTs.
> Coordinating control activities in interstate and inter-country borders.
> Collaboration with international organizations/

Outcomes:
> There is no expected decline in the prevalence of all diseases even after the implementation of the program.
> India has missed the December 2017 deadline announced for the elimination of Kala Azar (black fever) in 2017-18.
> Government efforts have resulted in an 86.45% decline in malaria cases and a 79.16% reduction in malaria-related deaths in 2021 as compared to 2015.

Programs under NVBDCP: Various programs under NVBDCP are:

1. **Kala-azar control program**: Kala-azar or visceral leishmaniasis (VL) is a chronic disease caused by an intracellular protozoan (Leishmania species) and transmitted to man by the bite of a female phlebotomus and fly. Currently, it is the main problem in Bihar, Jharkhand, West Bengal, and some parts of Uttar Pradesh.

   > It is a centrally sponsored program in endemic states from 1990-91. A tripartite MoU has been signed between India, Bangladesh, and Nepal for eradicating Kala Azar from the South East Asia region.

   > It has a target of reducing the annual incidence of Kala-Azar to less than 1 per 10000 population at the block PHC level.

2. **National Filaria Control Program**: *Bancroftian* filariasis caused by *Wuchereria bancrofti*, which is transmitted to man by the bites of infected mosquitoes *Culex, Anopheles, Mansonia*, and *Aedes*. Lymphatic filaria is prevalent in 18 states and union territories. Bancroftian filariasis is widely distributed while brugian filariasis caused by *Brugia malayi* is restricted to 6 states UP, Bihar, Andhra Pradesh, Orissa, Tamil Nadu, Kerala, and Gujarat.

   > The National Filaria Control Program was launched in 1955. It has the objective of controlling Lymphatic Filariasis in unsurveyed areas and urban areas through anti-parasitic and anti-larval measures.

   > The National Health Policy 2017 proposed the elimination of Lymphatic Filariasis and set the deadline for the disease's global eradication by 2020.

3. **Japanese Encephalitis Control Program**: Japanese encephalitis (JE) is a zoonotic disease caused by an Arbovirus, Flavivirus and transmitted by Culex mosquitoes. The Indian government organized a Japanese Encephalitis task team for early identification and case management.

4. **Dengue Control:** The program aims to control dengue outbreaks through surveillance, community participation particularly in the pre-monsoon period, and capacity building to ensure timely treatment.

Table 5.8 National Leprosy Eradication Program

<table>
<tr><td>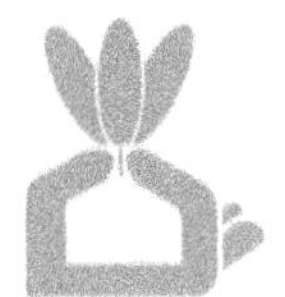</td><td>National Leprosy Eradication Program
Launched in 1954-55
Vision: leprosy free India by 2030</td></tr>
</table>

Goal: Provide free leprosy services to all parts of the population, including care for a disability the following cure through the integrated healthcare system

Objectives
- To reduce the prevalence rate to less than 1/10,000 population at the sub-national and district level
- To reduce Grade II disability % < 1 among new cases at the National level
- To reduce Grade II disability cases < 1 case per million population at the National level.
- Zero disabilities among new child cases.
- Zero stigma and discrimination against persons affected by leprosy

Functioning
- Providing leprosy health education to the local community.
- Leprosy diagnosis and care, including management of side effects.
- Self-care training for leprosy patients with ulcers.
- Counseling for leprosy patients to promote treatment compliance and disability prevention
- Leprosy Case Detection Campaigns (LCDC) in high-endemic districts for 14 days
- ASHA-based surveillance for suspected leprosy cases (ABSULS)
- Focused leprosy campaign (FLC) for case detection in low endemic districts
- Under the National Leprosy Eradication Program, the priority is early case detection, complete treatment of detected cases, and disease containment in close contact with index patients (persons diagnosed with leprosy).
- Active Case Detection and Regular Surveillance (ACDRS) in rural and urban areas to ensure early detection of leprosy cases to prevent Grade II disabilities.
- Convergence of leprosy screening programs under Rashtriya Bal Swasthya Karyakram (RBSK) for children (0-18 years) and Ayushman Bharat for people over 30 years of age
- NIKUSTH is a real-time leprosy reporting system implemented across India.
- To encourage district health functionaries, provision of certification, and awards to the districts for achieving leprosy elimination. There are two categories: 1) Gold Classification 2) Silver division
- Contact tracing is conducted, and Post Exposure Prophylaxis (PEP) with a single dose of Rifampicin (SDR) is administered to eligible contacts of the index case in order to break the transmission chain.
- Under the Disability Prevention and Medical Rehabilitation (DPMR) program, various services are provided, such as reaction management, MCR footwear, aids & appliances, and self-care kits.
- Reconstructive Surgeries (RCS) are conducted at District Hospitals/Medical Colleges/ Central Leprosy Institutes, and a welfare allowance of Rs 8000 is paid to each patient undergoing RCS.

Outcomes: In the year 2021-2022 the prevalence rate is 0.40 % as compared to 0.6; the percentage of child cases is 5.31% as compared to 9.04%t, and the annual case detection rate per 10000 is 4.71 as compared to 9.73 as it was in the year 2014-15.

Tuberculosis (TB) Control Program

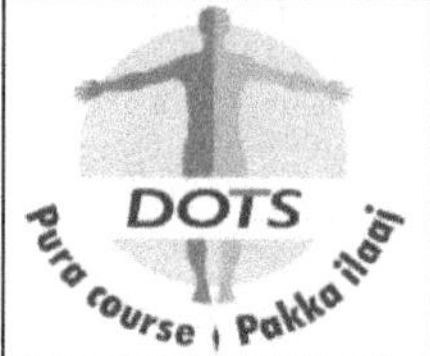

	Revised National TB Control Program (RNTCP)

Timeline of TB control programs in India:

- ➢ National TB Program **NTP** (1962-1997) started nationwide with a prime focus on BCG vaccinations as a preventive measure.

- ➢ A review of NTCP in 1992 resulted in the adoption of the RNTCP1993 in a phased manner by the Government of India in 1993 with the goal of decreasing the burden of TB till it ceases to be a public health problem.

- ➢ The pilot phase of RNTCP (1993-1996) was launched in a population of 2.4 million and was later expanded to cover 13 million people by 1995, 20 million by 1996, and the whole country by 2006.

- ➢ RNTCP phase-I began in 1997 with about 12% of population coverage and by March 2006, the whole country was brought under the program with the main focus on effective implementation of the DOTS strategy, which improves success rates and prevents MDR-TB.

- ➢ The focus of RNTCP Phase-II (2007-2011) was on the WHO **Stop TB Strategy**, which was linked to a TB-related MDG (combat HIV/AIDS, malaria, and other major infectious illnesses, including TB) and MDG target (halt and begin to reverse the incidence of TB by 2015). It also addressed MDG targets endorsed by the Stop TB Partnership, such as halving TB mortality and prevalence by 2015 compared to 1990, and eliminating TB by 2050, i.e. reducing incidence to 1 per million people.

- ➢ In line with this strategy, RNTCP India implemented all its **six principles** i.e. effectively pursuing DOTS, addressing TB-HIV enhanced package and MDR TB, strengthening the general health care system by deploying contractual staff, involving private practitioners and NGOs, empowering TB patients and communities through advocacy, communication and social mobilization (ACSM) and promoting research. As a result, the country's TB prevalence and fatality rates are on the decline.

- ➢ With the completion of RNTCP Phase-II, a newer plan was designed as National Strategic Plan (NSP) 2012-2017, which coincided with RNTCP Phase-III. The plan's vision was for a *"TB-free India."* The new goal was to provide all TB patients in the community with 'Universal Access' to high-quality diagnosis and treatment. This required maintaining the program's successes and expanding the reach and quality of care to all TB patients. **Six targets** to be achieved under Universal Access by 2015 were:

1. Early detection and treatment of at least 90% of estimated TB cases in the community, including HIV-associated TB; reduction of default rate below 5% in new cases and below 10% in retreatment cases,

2. Initial screening of all re-treatment smear-positive TB patients for drug-resistant TB and their management

3. HIV counseling and testing for all TB patients and linking HIV-infected TB patients to HIV care and support

4. Screening all persons attending HIV care and support facilities for TB

5. Successful treatment of at least 90% of all new TB patients, and at least 85% of all previously treated TB patients

6. Extending RNTCP services to patients diagnosed and treated in the private sector

Significant interventions and initiatives were taken during NSP 2012 - 2017 in terms of mandatory notification of all TB cases, integration of the program with the general health services, expansion of diagnostic services, programmatic management of drug-resistant TB, service expansion, single window service for TB/HIV cases, National drug resistance surveillance and revision of partnership guidelines.

Renaming of Revised National Tuberculosis Control Program (RNTCP)

➤ On January 1, 2020, India's TB control program got changed name. It is no longer known as the Revised National TB Control Program (RNTCP) and has been renamed the National Tuberculosis Elimination Program (NTEP).

➤ Eliminating TB by 2025: The change in name is in line with the larger goal of eliminating the disease by 2025, five years ahead of the Sustainable Development Goals target of 2030.

➤ The change in name is expected to give a "huge thrust to the people working for the elimination of tuberculosis from the top to bottom and the general population".

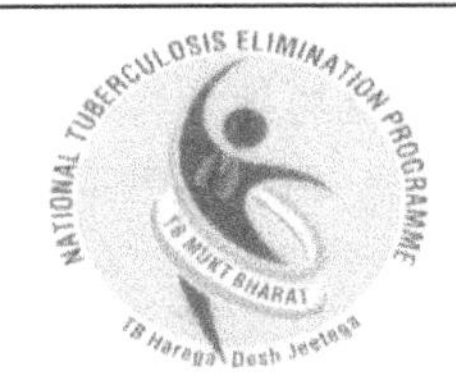

National Tuberculosis Elimination Program
Launched in 2020

To align with the ambitious goal, the program has been renamed from the Revised National Tuberculosis Control Program (RNTCP) to National Tuberculosis Elimination Program (NTEP). Its key features are:

➢ To address the socioeconomic determinants of TB while decreasing access barriers to diagnosis and treatment.

➢ All TB patients will receive nutritional support for the course of their treatment through the Nikshay Poshan Yojana.

➢ Rigorously working towards airborne infection control in hospital wards and outpatient waiting areas.

➢ Provision of chemoprophylaxis against TB disease in pediatric contacts of TB patients and People living with HIV (PLHIV).

➢ The process is ongoing for expanding TB preventive treatment for adult contacts too.

Nikshay Portal:

➢ **The Nikshay ecosystem:** It is the National TB information system which is a one-stop solution to manage information of patients and monitor program activity and performance throughout the country.

➢ **E-Nikshay platform**: It is the web-enabled patient management system for TB control under the National Tuberculosis Elimination Program (NTEP). It is developed and maintained by the Central TB Division (CTD), the Ministry of Health and Family Welfare in collaboration with the National Informatics Centre (NIC), and the World Health Organization.

➢ Nikshay Poshan Yojana (NPY): This scheme is aimed at providing financial support to TB patients for their nutrition. NHM provides financial support of rupees 500/month for nutritional support during the whole period of anti-TB therapy under this scheme.

➢ 'TB Mukt Bharat Abhiyaan' has been launched as a people's movement for TB elimination in India.

➢ India remains committed to supporting neighborhood countries with possible technical support and assistance.

➢ TB Harega Desh Jeetega Campaign: It was launched in September 2019 and showcases the highest level of commitment to the elimination of TB.

➢ The Saksham Project: It is a project of the Tata Institute of Social Sciences (TISS) that has been providing psycho-social counselling to Drug resistance TB patients.

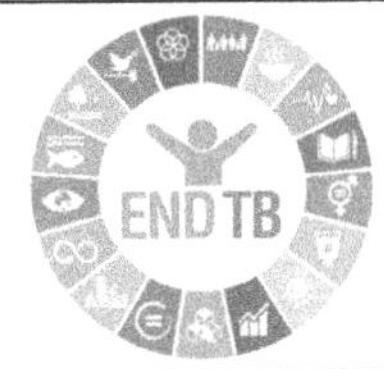 	**The National Strategic Plan for TB elimination** 2017 -2025

➢ The Prime Minister of India launched TB Free India campaign 'End TB Summit in Delhi on 13th March 2018

➢ The campaign calls for a social movement focused on patient-centric and holistic care driven by integrated actions for TB-free India

➢ Despite scaling up basic TB care in the public health system and treating more than 10 million TB patients under the RNTCP, the rate of decline is too slow to fulfill the 2030 SDG and 2035 End TB targets. This led to the adoption of NSP 2017-2025

➢ The NSP for TB elimination 2017–25 is a framework created by the Central TB Division, Ministry of Health and Family Welfare, in partnership with national and state governments, development partners, civil society organizations, and the corporate sector in India.

Vision, Goals, and Targets of NSP

Vision TB-Free India with zero deaths, disease, and poverty due to tuberculosis

Goal: To achieve a rapid decline in the burden of TB, morbidity, and mortality while working towards the elimination of TB in India by 2025.

Target: To quickly reduce TB cases in the country by 2030 in line with the global end TB targets and Sustainable Development Goals

National Strategic Plan for TB: Efforts to eradicate TB have resulted in an insufficient decrease in cases. To accelerate the rate of decline in TB incidence to more than 10-15% yearly, new interventions are necessary. According to the National strategic plan TB elimination has been combined with Detect – Treat – Prevent – Build (DTPB).

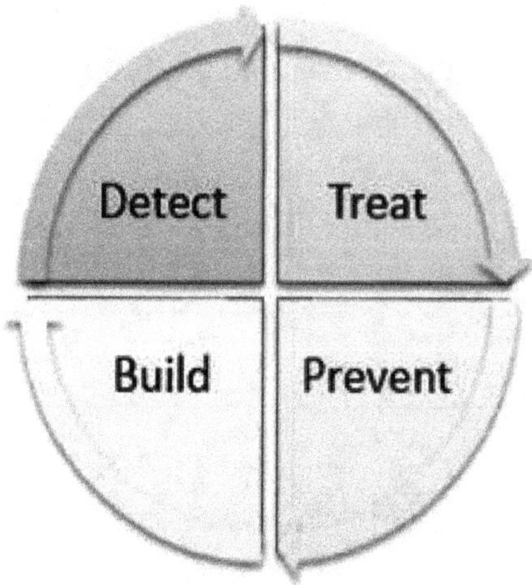

Detect: Early identification of suspected TB cases at the first point of care (private or public) and fast diagnosis utilizing high-sensitivity diagnostic tests to provide universal access to quality TB diagnosis, including drug-resistant TB. The DTPB approach and the steps to implement are:

Table 5.9 DTPB Approach

Detect	Steps
Find all DS-TB (drug-sensitive) and DRTB (drug-resistant) cases, focusing on TB patients receiving private care and undiagnosed TB in high-risk populations.	➤ Free, high-sensitivity diagnostic tests ➤ Effective approaches to involve private providers ➤ Universal testing for drug-resistant TB ➤ Systematic screening of high-risk populations
Treat	**Steps**
Initiate and sustain all patients on appropriate anti-TB treatment wherever they seek care, with patient-friendly systems and social support.	➤ Free TB drugs for all TB cases ➤ Universal daily regimen with fixed dose combinations for TB cases and rapid scale-up of short-course regimens for drug-resistant TB ➤ Patient-friendly adherence monitoring and social support to sustain TB treatment ➤ Elimination of excessive costs by linkage of eligible TB patients with social welfare schemes including nutritional support
Prevent	**Steps**
Prevent the emergence of TB in susceptible populations	➤ Step up airborne infection control measures ➤ Strengthen contact investigation ➤ Preventive treatment in high-risk groups ➤ Manage latent TB infections ➤ Address social determinants of disease

Table 5.9 *Contd...*

Build	Steps
Build and strengthen policies, Empower institutions and human resources with enhanced capacities. Private sector participation to improve efficiency	➢ Dedicated staff for TB surveillance network in the country ➢ Scale up technical assistance at national and state levels. ➢ Build supportive structures for surveillance, research, and innovations. ➢ Strengthen RNTCP (revised national TB control program) regulatory capacity to control TB drugs through appropriate laws, regulations, and policies ➢ Position TB on the health and development agenda to ensure enough resources.

National AIDS Control Program (NACP)

In 1986, India found its first case of AIDS. In 1992, it started the National AIDS and STD Control Program (NACP). 35 years since then, NACP has gone through five different stages to become one of the largest programs in the world.

1. The first phase of the NACP (1992-1999) focused on awareness generation and blood safety.

2. The second phase (1999-2007) witnessed the launch of direct interventions across the prevention-detection-treatment continuum with capacity building of States on program management.

3. The third phase (2007-2012) was the story of scale-up with program management decentralized up to the district level.

4. The fourth phase (2012-2017) was a period of consolidation and enhanced Government funding.

5. The NACP Phase-IV (Extension) was first approved for the period of 2017-2020 and then further extended for one more year i.e., 2020-21.

Table 5.10 Timeline of AIDS control Programs and their features

Program	Salient features
Initial National HIV/AIDS responses (1985-1991)	➢ Constitution of National AIDS Committee ➢ Focus on blood screening and awareness generation
NACP Phase-I (1992-1999)	➢ Establishment of the National Aids Control Board, (NACB), National Aids Control Organization (NACO), and State Aids Prevention and Control Societies (SACS)

Table 5.10 *Contd...*

Program	Salient features
	➢ Implementation of large-scale awareness generation campaigns ➢ Licensing of blood banks and banning of professional donors ➢ Collaboration with non-profit organizations (NGO)/community-based organizations (CBO) for prevention interventions among high-risk groups (HRG) ➢ Expansion of surveillance networks
NACP Phase-II (1999-2007)	➢ Launch and expansion of targeted interventions (TI) through NGO/CBO ➢ Establishment of facilities for voluntary counseling and testing (VCT) and perinatal transmission (PPTCT) ➢ Introduction of antiretrovirals agents (ARV) and establishment of ART centers ➢ Constitution of the National Council on AIDS
NACP Phase-III (2007-2012)	➢ Rapid scale-up of the service delivery facilities pan India ➢ Offering HIV counseling and testing services to pregnant women as an essential component of antenatal services ➢ The transition of donor-funded interventions for the key population ➢ Decentralization of HIV programs i.e. involving states and communities
NACP Phase-IV (2012-2017)	➢ Increased funding by the Government of India providing 73% of the total budget for NACP ➢ Launch of National HIV/AIDS toll-free helpline 1097 ➢ Adoption of dual elimination of vertical transmission (of HIV & Syphilis) in NACP guidelines ➢ Launch of NACP interventions in prisons and other closed settings ➢ Introduction of HIV and AIDS (Prevention and Control) in the Rajya Sabha ➢ Mid-term review of NACP Phase-IV
NACP Phase-IV Extension (2017-21)	➢ Launch and scale up 'Test and Treat policy for HIV patients ➢ 'Mission Sampark' to trace those who are left to follow up and are to be brought under ART (antiretroviral therapy) ➢ Launch of differentiated care (DSDM) to strengthen follow-up adherence and retention of HIV patients ➢ Scale-up of NACP interventions in prisons and other closed settings ➢ Development and roll-out of patient-centric, IT-enabled monitoring, evaluation, and surveillance system with embedded supply chain management ➢ Third-party evaluation of NACP Phase-IV and Extension ➢ Ensuring uninterrupted service delivery to targeted beneficiaries during Covid 19

NACP-IV Extension

The targets for NACP-IV extension were to ensure:

- More than 99% of the population will be kept HIV-free
- More than 70 lakh of the key population is to be covered annually through a comprehensive HIV prevention program.
- Around 15 crores of a vulnerable population (including five crores of pregnant women) will be tested for HIV within three years of the project.
- Two crores thirty-two lakh (2,32,00,000) units of blood will be collected at NACO's supported blood banks during the three years of the project
- Two crores eighty-two lakh episodes of sexually transmitted infections will be managed under the project for three years of duration
- Seventeen lakhs of PLHIV will be put on free anti-retroviral treatment by the end of the project period.

Achievements of Phase IV and Phase IV Extension

In India, there were an estimated 23.49 lakh (2.35 million) People Living with HIV (PLHIV), with an adult HIV prevalence of 0.22% in 2019. Children living with HIV comprised 3.4% of the total PLHIV estimates. HIV-infected women constituted around 44% of the total estimated 15+ years PLHIV.

From 2012-13 to 2019-20 total collection of blood across the country has increased by 170 folds. There were 69.22 thousand new HIV infections in 2019 which has declined by 37% since 2010. There were 59000 AIDS-related deaths in 2019, which has declined by 66% since 2010. This rate of decline in India is much better than the global average of 23% decline in new HIV infections and a 39% decline in AIDS-related deaths.

Table 5.11 National Aids Control Program (NACP) PHASE V

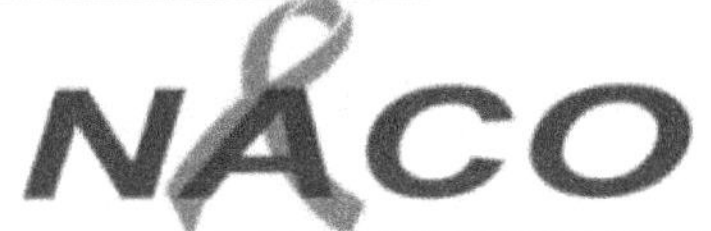	**NACP PHASE-V (2021-26)** Paving the way for an AIDS-Free India
Achieving zero new infections, zero AIDS-related deaths, and zero discrimination	
Goals: ➢ Reduce new infections by 80% by 2024 (Baseline 2010) ➢ Reduce AIDS-related mortality by 80% ➢ Eliminate vertical transmission of HIV ➢ Promote universal access to quality services ➢ Eliminate HIV/AIDS-related stigma and discrimination.	

Table 5.11 *Contd...*

Objectives:

➢ To achieve 95–95–95 testing and treatment targets within all age groups.

➢ 95% of women of reproductive age have their HIV and sexual and reproductive health service needs met; 95% of pregnant and breastfeeding women living with HIV have suppressed viral loads, and 95% of HIV-exposed children are tested by 2025

➢ 95% of people at risk of HIV infection use appropriate and effective prevention options

➢ Less than 10% of people living with HIV experience stigma and discrimination

Expected outcomes:

➢ It will support the national AIDS and STD response to achieve Sustainable Development Goal 3.3 of ending the HIV/AIDS epidemic as a public health issue by 2030 through prevention, detection, and treatment services.

➢ Around 8 crores of people will be covered annually with a tailored package of prevention-detection-treatment services

➢ More than 99.5% of the adult population will be kept HIV-free.

➢ Around 27 crore HIV tests will be undertaken, including around 14 crores among pregnant women, in five years of NACP Phase-V.

➢ Twenty-one lakh HIV-infected people will be on Antiretroviral Treatment (ART) by the end of the projected period.

➢ Around 80 lakh viral load tests will be conducted on ART HIV-infected people to monitor the effectiveness of treatment towards the attainment of viral load suppression.

➢ The program will offer free HIV prevention, detection, and treatment services in facility and community settings to high-risk, vulnerable, and other 'at-risk' populations and people living with HIV, promoting equity and inclusiveness.

➢ The program promotes a decentralized method of program monitoring at the district level based on community input.

HIV and AIDS (Prevention and Control) Act, 2017

➢ The HIV and AIDS (Prevention and Control) Act, 2017 is landmark legislation. The Act aims to address stigma and discrimination so that those infected with and affected by HIV and AIDS are not discriminated against in their homes, workplaces, and healthcare settings.

➢ The Act also restores the constitutional, legislative, and human rights of people affected by AIDS. It also provides a grievance redressal mechanism in the form of a complaints officer at each establishment and an Ombudsman at the state level.

Reproductive, Maternal, Neonatal, Child, and Adolescent Health

1. Janani Suraksha Yojana (JSY)
2. Pradhan Mantri Surakshit Matritva Abhiyan (PMSMA)

3. Navjaat Shishu Suraksha Karyakram (NSSK)
4. Janani Shishu Suraksha Karyakaram (JSSK)
5. Rashtriya Kishor Swasthya Karyakram (RKSK)
6. Universal immunization program (UIP)
7. Family planning program (FP)

Table 5.12 Janani Suraksha Yojana

जननी सुरक्षा योजना	**Janani Suraksha Yojana (JSY)** Launched on 12th April 2005
Goal To reduce maternal and infant mortality rates among economically weaker women by encouraging institutional deliveries.	
Objectives	➢ The program promotes institutional delivery among low-income pregnant women to reduce mother and newborn mortality. ➢ To provide medical facilities and financial assistance to pregnant women. ➢ During institutional deliveries, women and newborns can be saved from pregnancy-related deaths due to the availability of skilled doctors, nurses, and pediatricians
Functioning	➢ It is a center-funded scheme. The JSY yojna provides medical facilities and financial assistance to pregnant women. ➢ In order to give birth to only two children, all the medical and financial facilities for pregnant women will be provided by the government under this Janani Suraksha Yojana 2021 ➢ Under this scheme, pregnant women from both rural and urban areas of the country can get themselves registered. ➢ The yojana has identified ASHA, (the accredited social health activist) and anganwadi workers as a link between the Government and poor women. ➢ Financial assistance will be provided by the government to pregnant women only when they are 19 years of age or more ➢ Every beneficiary registered under the scheme must have MCH card as well as Janani Suraksha Yojana card. ➢ Identification of complicated cases and 3 antenatal and post-natal visits ➢ After the delivery, information is sent to the mother and child about free vaccination for five years ➢ The pregnant females enrolled under JYS have to go to government hospitals or any private institute which is selected by the government
Outcomes	Through this scheme, the government will not only reduce the mortality rate of mothers but will also reduce the death of children. With this, poor women can avoid emergency situations and get safe delivery.

Table 5.13 Pradhan Mantri Surakshit Matritva Abhiyan

	Pradhan Mantri Surakshit Matritva Abhiyan (PMSMA) Launched on 31st July 2016
Objectives	The program was launched with an aim to provide fixed-day assured, comprehensive, and quality antenatal care universally to all pregnant women (in 2nd and 3rd trimester) on the 9th of every month.
Functioning	➤ The beneficiaries are first registered in Pradhan Mantri Surakshit Matritva Abhiyan (PMSMA). ➤ After registration, all basic laboratory investigations are done by ANM & staff nurses then examined by the Medical Officer. ➤ Identification for high-risk status (like anemia, gestational diabetes, hypertension, infection, etc.) is done based on lab investigations e.g. ultrasound, Hb, urine albumin, rapid malaria test, blood grouping, CBC ESR, etc.
Outcomes	Access to quality antenatal services during pregnancy helps to detect life-threatening complications during childbirth.

Table 5.14 Navjaat Shishu Suraksha Karyakram

	Navjaat Shishu Suraksha Karyakram (NSSK) Launched in November 2020
Objectives	The program aims to have a trained health professional at every delivery point. The 2-day training will cut neonatal mortality in the country. Some training activities include prevention of hypothermia, prevention of infection, early initiation of breastfeeding, and basic new-born resuscitation

Table 5.14 *Contd...*

Functioning	➢ Creation of newborn care units at district level hospitals, stabilization units at the community health center level, and newborn corners at the primary health center level to provide specialized care by trained staff and doctors. ➢ Skill development of ASHAs and skilled birth attendants to ensure home-based newborn and child care. ➢ Ensuring availability of pediatricians at community health center level hospitals
Outcomes	This initiative could cut newborn mortality, which accounts for 45% of under-5 mortality.

Table 5.15 Janani Shishu Suraksha Karyakaram

	Janani Shishu Suraksha Karyakaram (JSSK) Launched in November, 2011
Objectives	To eliminate out-of-pocket expenses for both pregnant women and sick infants accessing public health institutions for treatment.
Functioning	➢ Entitlement of pregnant women to a wide range of benefits like C-sections, medications and consumables, diagnostics, free meals while in the hospital, and cashless delivery all included in the program. Exemption from user fees, free transportation to and from health care facilities, etc. ➢ Free entitlements for sick newborns till 30 days after birth ➢ Periodic reviews and field visits are undertaken at various levels to assess the implementation of Janani Shishu Suraksha Karyakram (JSSK) by the States. ➢ Since the launch of JSSK, nine Common Review Missions (CRMs) have been undertaken.

Table 5.15 *Contd...*

Outcomes	➢ Policy making and the spread of information on entitlements have started in all states.
	➢ The awareness about the entitlements of pregnant women under the JSSK scheme has improved.
	➢ The JSSK entitlements for pregnant women and sick infants up to one year of age are operational across all states, resulting in a considerable reduction in out-of-pocket expenditures.
	➢ Free drugs, diagnostics, diet, and assured home-to-facility transport as well as drop back have improved across all the states.
	➢ OPD and Inpatient department IPD services are provided free of cost to all pregnant beneficiaries in all the states.
	➢ The provision for free diagnostic facilities, including basic lab tests, for pregnant women, has improved significantly in most of states.
	➢ Provision for blood for pregnant women and sick infants is available at all the District hospitals visited.
	➢ Free diet is being provided to pregnant beneficiaries in most of the States

Table 5.16 Rashtriya Kishor Swasthya Karyakram (RKSK)

RKSK	Rashtriya Kishor Swasthya Karyakram (RKSK)
Goal	The program vision enables all adolescents in India to realize their full potential by making informed and responsible decisions related to their health and well-being and by accessing the services and support
Objective	➢ Improve nutrition: To reduce the prevalence of malnutrition and iron-deficiency anemia in adolescent girls and boys
	➢ Improve sexual and reproductive health (SRH): To improve knowledge, attitudes, and relation to SRH. To reduce teenage pregnancies, improve birth preparedness, and complications, readiness and provide early parenting support for adolescent parents
	➢ Enhance mental health: Address mental health concerns of adolescents

Table 5.16 *Contd...*

	➢ Prevent injuries and violence: Promote favorable attitudes for preventing injuries and violence (including GBV) among adolescents ➢ Prevent substance misuse: Increase adolescent awareness of the adverse effects and consequences of substance misuse ➢ Address NCDs: Promote behavior change in adolescents to prevent NCDs such as hypertension, stroke, cardiovascular diseases and diabetes
Functioning	➢ Strategies/interventions to achieve objectives can be broadly grouped as: • Community-based Education (PE) • Quarterly Adolescent Health Day (AHD) • Weekly Iron and Folic Acid Supplementation Program (WIFS) • Menstrual Hygiene Scheme (MHS) ➢ Facility-based interventions: Strengthening of Adolescent Friendly Health Clinics (AFHC)
Outcomes	During clinic sessions, adolescents, married and unmarried, girls and boys, receive preventative, promotive, curative, and counseling treatments, as well as routine check-ups at the primary, secondary, and tertiary levels of care

Universal immunization Program

Immunization against preventable childhood diseases is the right of every child. In view of providing this right, the Government of India launched the Universal Immunization Program (UIP) in 1985, one of the largest health programs of its kind in the world. Today Immunization division is a part of the Reproductive Child Healthcare (RCH) program under the National Health Mission (NHM)

Table 5.17 Evolution of the immunization Program in India

Year	Program
1978	Launch of a National immunization program called Expanded Program of immunization (EPI) with the introduction of vaccines: BCG, OPV, DPT, and typhoid vaccines
1980-81	Introduction of Tetanus to school children
1981-82	BCG inoculation initially included under the National Tuberculosis Control Program in 1962 was brought under EPI
1981	The typhoid-paratyphoid vaccine dropped from EPI in 1981
1983	Tetanus toxoid vaccine for pregnant women was added in EPI in 1983
1985	Introduction of Universal Immunization Program (UIP) by ending EPI ➢ Indigenous vaccine production capacity enhanced ➢ Cold chain established

Table 5.17 *Contd...*

	➢ Phased implementation - all districts covered by 1989-90. ➢ Monitoring and evaluation system implemented ➢ Vaccination against Measles introduced
1986	➢ Universal Immunization Program renamed as National Technology Mission ➢ India attained self-sustainability in vaccine production.
1990	Added Vitamin-A supplement to immunization program in 1990
1992	UIP became part of Child Survival and Safe Motherhood (CSSM)
1997	Launching of Reproductive Child health program which included both UIP and child health program
2005	National Rural Health Mission
2012	➢ The Government of India declared 2012 as the Year of intensification of routine immunization ➢ Strategy to reach all children including migrants in remote inaccessible backward areas and urban slums
2014	Mission Indradhanush

Mission Indradhanush (2014)

- It was launched in 2014 to fully immunize more than 89 lakh children who are either unvaccinated or partially vaccinated under UIP.

- It provides vaccination against 12 Vaccine-Preventable Diseases (VPD) i.e. diphtheria, whooping cough, tetanus, polio, tuberculosis, hepatitis B, rubella, measles, poliomyelitis meningitis, pneumonia, Human papillomavirus (HPV), Haemophilus influenza B infections, Japanese encephalitis (JE)

- However, vaccination against Japanese Encephalitis and Haemophilus influenza are being provided in selected districts of the country

- Under MI, all vaccines are provided as per National Immunization Schedule.

Stages of Intensified Mission Indradhanush

Intensified Mission Indradhanush 1.0: This mission was launched in 2017, to further intensify the immunization program.

> ➢ It aims to reach every child aged under two years and pregnant women who were left uncovered under the routine immunization program.

> ➢ Under this mission, greater focus was given to urban areas which were left under the mission Indradhanush.

Intensified Mission Indradhanush 2.0:

> ➢ It was a nationwide immunization campaign to commemorate the 25th anniversary of the Pulse Polio Program (2019-20).

➢ The aim was to ensure reaching the unreached with all available vaccines and accelerate the coverage of children and pregnant women in identified districts and blocks.

➢ It had full immunization coverage targets in 272 districts spread across 27 States.

Intensified Mission Indradhanush 3.0 (2021)

➢ The focus was on children and pregnant women who missed their vaccine doses during the COVID-19 pandemic.

Table 5.18 Intensified Mission Indradhanush

	Intensified Mission Indradhanush Launched in 2021
Goal To ensure full immunization with all available vaccines for children up to 2 years of age and pregnant women	
Objective	➢ To strengthen the health system for immunization program ➢ Increase demand and reduce barriers for people to access immunization services through improved social mobilization ➢ Improve program service delivery for equitable and efficient immunization services by all districts. ➢ Strengthen and maintain a robust surveillance system for vaccine Preventable Diseases (VPDs) and Adverse Events Following Immunization (AEFI) ➢ Introduce and expand the use of new and underutilized vaccines and technology in UIP. ➢ Contribute to the global eradication of polio and measles, elimination of maternal and neonatal tetanus, and control and prevention of rubella
Functioning	➢ Identify areas that are left out, drop out, and develop strategies ➢ Identify community representatives who could support in reaching the specific communities with messages ➢ Focussing on identified high-risk populations with traditionally low coverage, such as slum dwellers, nomadic populations, and migrant families living in brick kilns and construction sites ➢ Implementing Rapid Immunization Skill Enhancement (RISE) – a continuous knowledge-building system ➢ Effective communication and social mobilization activities (mass media, interpersonal communication, school and youth networks, and corporates

Table 5.18 *Contd...*

	➢ Creation of enabling environment to generate confidence in vaccines ➢ Deployment of ANMs to areas outside her own sub-center and block with weak immunization coverage ➢ Engaging all ANMs in the district for a need-based 7-day plan ➢ Integration of the Health and Family Welfare Department with the Education Department to link vaccination distribution with other health treatments such as WIFS (Weekly iron-folic acid supplements) and deworming for school-age children, with the goal of increasing coverage and lowering delivery costs. ➢ Support state in identifying essential activities and their inclusion in state project implementation plans
Outcome	➢ During the various phases of Mission Indradhanush, a total of 3.86 crore children and 96.8 lakh pregnant women have been vaccinated. ➢ The first two phases of Mission Indradhanush resulted in a 6.7% increase in full immunization coverage in a year. ➢ The Full immunization coverage among children aged 12-23 months of age has increased from 62% (NFHS-4) to 76.4% (NFHS-5).

Table 5.19 Family Planning

जोड़ी ज़िम्मेदार जो प्लान करे परिवार	**Family Planning Program** Launched in 1952

Goals
To achieve population stabilization goals and ensure universal access to:
   ➢ Sexual and reproductive health care services STD/HIV prevention
   ➢ Safe pregnancy
   ➢ Breastfeeding
   ➢ Women's nutrition
   ➢ Adolescent reproductive health	

Objectives	➢ Making population stabilization a national priority ➢ To increase access to spacing methods with a specific focus on improving intrauterine devices (IUD) utilization. ➢ Addressing social determinants of health such as age at marriage ➢ To strengthen the quality of care, including counseling services, ➢ To increase the contraceptive prevalence rate among eligible couples ➢ To increase access of prospective clients for terminal family planning methods, especially in pockets of higher order birth.

Table 5.19 *Contd...*

	➢ To implement a State-specific policy, which covers the availability of safe abortion services and emergency contraception at all levels of health care. ➢ To reduce infant and maternal morbidity and mortality ➢ Increasing budgetary allocations for family planning ➢ To improve the safety and efficacy of family welfare services.
Functioning	➢ Improving operative and post-operative care practices to bring down morbidity and mortality due to sterilization. ➢ Ensuring an uninterrupted supply of essential drugs, vaccines, and contraceptives, adequate in quantity and appropriate in quality. ➢ Home distribution of contraceptives by ASHA workers ➢ Engaging men and women in recognizing their reproductive health ➢ Organizing IUD insertion camps at the PHC level on immunization day ➢ Making available emergency contraceptives in all CHCs and PHCs ➢ Social marketing of condoms, oral pills, and contraceptive devices ➢ Ensuring the availability of trained doctors for abortions
Outcome	The total fertility rate has declined to 2 from 2.2 as the contraceptive prevalence rate has increased to 67% as compared to 54%. Institutional births have increased to 88% i.e 9% more as compared to 79%.

National Nutritional Programs:

1. National Iodine Deficiency Disorders Control Program
2. MAA (Mothers' Absolute Affection) Program for Infant and Young Child Feeding
3. Intensified National Iron Plus Initiative for Anemia Control
4. Integrated Child Development Services (ICDS)
5. Mid-Day Meal Program

Table 5.20 National Iodine Deficiency Disorders Control Program

सही आयोडीन नमक की पहचान आयोडीन नमक	**National Iodine Deficiency Disorders Control Program** Launched in 1992
Goal	To bring the prevalence of IDD to below 5% in the country and to ensure 100% consumption of adequately iodized salt (15ppm) at the household level.

Table 5.20 *Contd...*

Objectives	To enhance the production, demand, and supply of iodized salt and ban the sale of non-iodized salt for direct human consumption in the entire country.
Functioning	➢ Surveys to assess the magnitude of the Iodine deficiency disorders. ➢ Supply iodized salt in place of common salt. ➢ Resurvey after every 5 years to assess the extent of Iodine deficiency disorders and the impact of iodized salt. ➢ Laboratory monitoring of iodized salt and urinary iodine excretion. ➢ Health education and publicity
Outcomes	➢ The consumption of adequately iodized salt at the household level has increased from 51.1% (as per NFHS III report 2005-06) to 71.1% (as per CES report, 2009). ➢ Over the years the Total Goiter Rate (TGR) in the entire country is reduced significantly. ➢ Production of iodized salt in the country reached 65.00 lakh MT which is adequate to meet the requirement of the population.

Table 5.21 Intensified National iron plus initiative (I-NIPI) for Anaemia Control

	Intensified National iron plus initiative (I-NIPI) for Anaemia Control Launched in 2019		
Goal	To reduce the prevalence/burden of anemia in India by 3 percentage points per annum		
Objectives	Decrease anemia prevalence by 18% in all targets by 2022		
Functioning	I-NIPI popularly known as Anemia Mukt Bharat (AMB) program, works upon the 6x6x6 strategy to combat anemia, i.e 6 beneficiaries, 6 interventions, and 6 institutional mechanisms. Further emphasis is on Test, Treat and Talk camps.		
	Six beneficiaries	Six key interventions	Six Institutional Mechanism
	➢ Children. ➢ Adolescent girls and boys. ➢ Women of reproductive age. ➢ Pregnant women ➢ Lactating mothers	➢ Prophylactic iron and folic acid supplementation; ➢ Deworming. ➢ Intensified year-round behavior change	➢ Intra-ministerial coordination ➢ Strengthening supply chain and logistics ➢ National center of excellence and

Table 5.21 Contd...

		communication campaign ➤ ensuring delayed cord clamping in new-borns to increase hemoglobin in pre-term babies ➤ Testing of anemia using digital methods ➤ Mandatory provision of iron and folic acid fortified foods in government-funded health programs. ➤ Addressing non-nutritional causes of anemia ➤ Specified doses and schedules of Iron folic acid syrup/ tablets	advanced research on anemia control ➤ National Anemia Mukt Bharat unit ➤ Anemia Mukt Bharat digital portal
	Iron folic acid syrup/tablets are provided for free to all by anganwadis or government hospitals.		
Outcomes	We are expecting better outcomes than before as in 2016, the percent decrease in deficiency was found to be between 0.1% and 1.1% over a 10-year period, which is quite low and indicates that the program must be strengthened and refocused.		

Table 5.22 Mid-day meal scheme

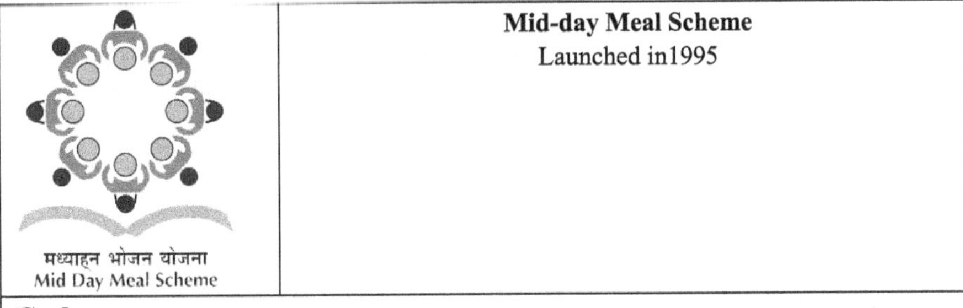 	**Mid-day Meal Scheme** Launched in1995
Goal To increase school attendance and enrolments, to decrease the school dropout rate along with the beneficial impact on children's nutrition	

Table 5.22 *Contd...*

Objectives	1. To increase the enrolment of the children belonging to disadvantaged sections in the schools. 2. Leading enrolment to increased attendance in the schools. 3. To retain children studying in classes 1-8. 4. To provide nutritional support to the children in the elementary stage in drought-affected areas.
Functioning	It is implemented using one of the three models: 1. Decentralized model – Preparing meals on the site by local cooks, 2. Centralized model – In the place of local on-site cooks, under this model, an external organization cooks food and delivers it to the schools. 3. International assistance – Various international charity organizations aid government schools.
	Other features: ➢ The schools procure AGMARK quality items for the preparation of midday meals. ➢ The meals are to be served on the school premises only. ➢ Each school should have a hygienic cooking infrastructure to cook mid-day meals ➢ The School Management Committee (SMCs) plays a vital role in the monitoring of MDMS. ➢ Principals are empowered to utilize the school funds on the account of midday meal fund exhaustion. However, the same has to be reimbursed to the midday meal fund as soon as the school is credited with the MDM fund. ➢ The state's Food and Drug Administration Department may collect samples to check the nutritional value and quality of the meals. ➢ Food allowance is to be provided to the children whenever cooked meals are not provided due to unforeseen circumstances. The allowance is calculated according to • Quantity of food grains as per entitlement of the child • Cooking costs prevail in the State.
Outcomes	It is found that the midday meal scheme was associated with 13-32% of India's improvement in height-for-age z-scores (HAZ) between 2006 and 2016. The prevalence of stunting was significantly lower in areas where the mid scheme was implemented in 2005

Recent modifications in Mid-day Meal Scheme to PM POSHAN

In September 2021, the Mid-Day Meal Scheme was renamed "PM POSHAN" or Pradhan Mantri Poshan Shakti Nirman. This scheme would provide hot-cooked meals to pre-primary, government, and government-aided primary schools. The modified scheme has been launched for 5 years, from 2021-22 to 2025-26, with a budget of 1,30,794.90 crore. The government hopes it will benefit 11.80 crore children studying in 11.20 lakh schools across India.

The scheme is different from the mid-day meal scheme in the following ways:

1. Apart from providing nutritional meals to schoolchildren, the revised scheme will also focus on monitoring the nutritional levels of schoolchildren.

2. A nutritional expert will be appointed in each school to ensure that the BMI, weight levels, and hemoglobin levels of the students are monitored.

3. In districts with a high prevalence of anemia, special provisions for nutritional items would be made.

4. The government is also considering developing nutrition gardens on school campuses with active participation by students.

5. There could also be cooking competitions held under the scheme to promote traditional food and innovative menus based on local ingredients.

Table 5.23 Integrated Child Development Services Scheme

	Integrated Child Development Services Scheme Launched in1975
I.C.D.S	
Goal	ICDS is one of the largest national development programs in the world, It targets 7 million women between the ages of 16 and 44, 7 million pregnant and nursing mothers, and over 34 million children aged 0 to 6 years. The scheme is aimed to improve the health, nutrition and education of the target community.
Objectives	➢ To improve the health and nutritional status of children 0–6 years and pregnant and lactating mothers. ➢ To reduce the incidence of their mortality and school dropout ➢ To provide a firm foundation for proper psychological, physical and social development of the child. ➢ To enhance the capability of the mother to look after the normal health and nutritional needs of the child ➢ To facilitate, educate and empower adolescent girls so as to enable them to become self-reliant and aware citizens. ➢ To achieve effective policy and implementation coordination among various departments and programs aimed to promote child development

Table 5.23 Contd...

Functioning	Integrated Child Development Services is centrally-sponsored and will provide the following six services to the beneficiaries: ➢ **Supplementary Nutrition (SNP)**: Supplementary feeding and growth monitoring services ➢ **Health & Nutrition Check-Up**: regular health check-ups, treatment of diarrhea, deworming, weight recording, immunizations, and distribution of simple medicines. ➢ **Immunization:** Vaccination for VPDs diphtheria, polio, pertussis, measles, TB ,and tetanus. ➢ **Non-Formal Education for Children in Pre-School**: It prepares young children for primary school and frees older siblings (especially girls) to attend school. ➢ **Health and Nutrition Education**: The women in the age group of 15-45 years are enabled to look after their own health, nutrition, and development needs as well as that of their children and families. ➢ **Referral Services**: Anganwadi workers are trained to detect disabilities and diseases in children requiring immediate medical attention and refer them to a hospital or primary health center for early intervention.
Outcomes	➢ There are presently 5652 ICDS projects functional in the country comprising 4533 in rural, 759 in tribal, and 360 in urban areas. ➢ Different services are delivered in an integrated manner to ensure the beneficiary's right to survival, growth, protection, and development. ➢ The ICDS services have a positive impact on promoting institutional delivery in rural India. Now expectant mothers are receiving correct counseling from ICDS, and understand the health risks of non-institutional deliveries.

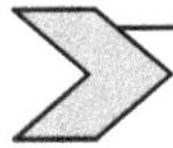

CHAPTER 6

Role of Pharmacist in Disaster Management

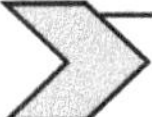

6.0 Introduction

This chapter aims to provide students with an understanding of the following topics
- Various types of disasters and their management.
- Role of pharmacist in disaster management

A disaster is an event that occurs suddenly and unexpectedly and has the potential to cause serious harm to mankind.

Disaster causes disruption to the human, social, economic, and ecological life of society. It causes disruption, death, damage, destruction, disability, epidemic, diversion of resources and immense financial burden to the Government.

According to Disaster Management Act

"Disaster is a catastrophe, mishap, calamity, or grave occurrence in any area arising from natural or man-made causes, or by accident or negligence which results in substantial loss of life or human suffering, damage to, and destruction of property, or damage to, or degradation to environment and is of such a nature and magnitude as to be beyond the coping capacity of the community of the affected area".

The extent of injuries and losses to humans depends on the nature and type of disasters.

Classification of disasters

A. Natural Disasters

> **Predictable disasters:** Some disasters like cyclones, floods, and droughts can be fairly predicted.

> **Unpredictable sudden disasters**: Earthquakes, landslides, flashfloods, and tsunamis often occur suddenly.

➤ **Biological disasters**: These involve disease, disability, or death on a large scale among humans, animals, and plants due to microorganisms like bacteria, viruses, fungi, and their toxins.

B. Man-made disasters: Riots, accidents, fires, industrial accidents, ecological disasters like environmental pollution and degradation, and technological disasters.

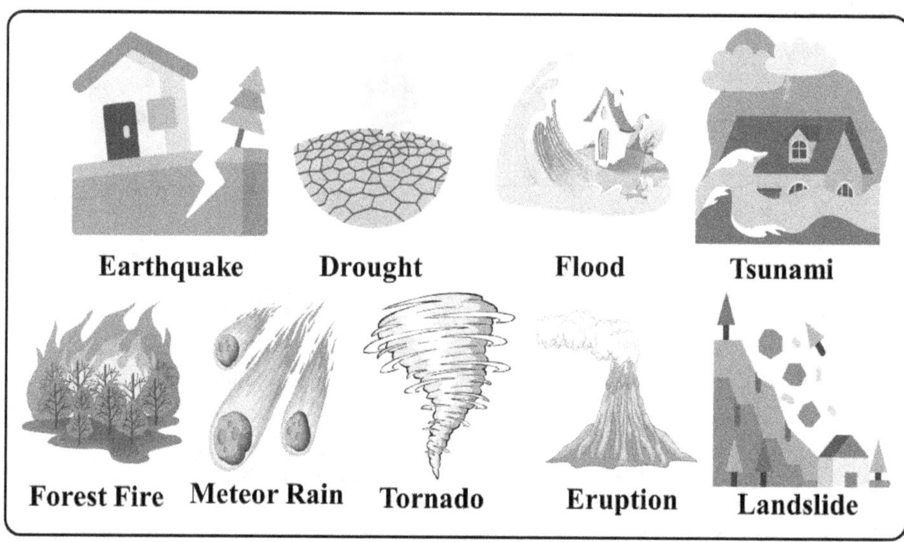

(a) Natural disasters

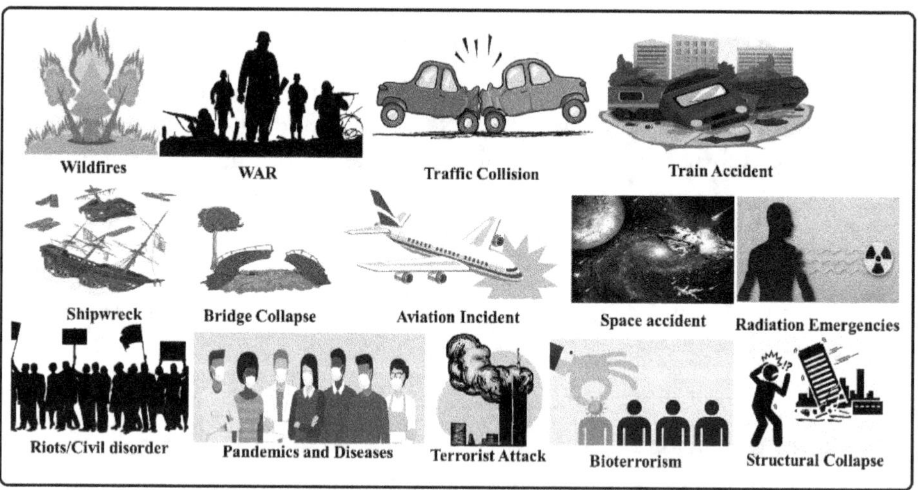

(b) Man-made disasters

Figure 6.1 Types of Disasters

Disaster Management: Disasters have increased in frequency, intensity, and scale today. They cause irreparable damages in terms of deaths and injuries. Disaster management aims to prevent deaths, diseases and injuries emerging from any kind of disaster.

Public health disaster is a situation in which the need for health/medical care exceeds the immediately available resources, and in which urgent extraordinary and coordinating measures are necessary to maintain normal quality standards.

Phases of Disaster Management: Four important steps have to be taken to mitigate the adverse consequences of disasters and to provide comprehensive and definitive medical care to the disaster victims. These are:

➢ **Prevention** of the disaster effects

➢ **Preparedness** for meeting emergencies

➢ Well laid down and practiced system of **Response**

➢ Planned system of short-term and long-term **Recovery** and **Rehabilitation**.

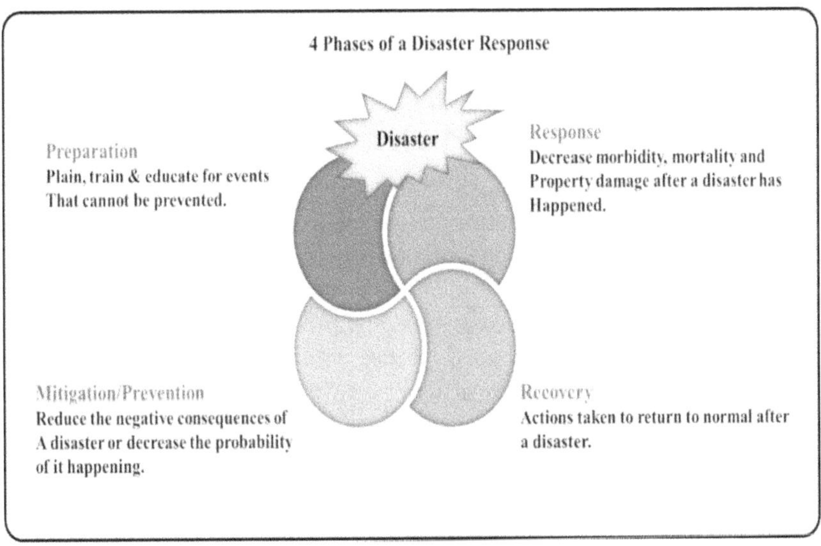

Figure 6.2 PPRR cycle- Four phases of disaster management

The PPRR cycle will involve a multidisciplinary system of planning for disasters and requires the medical and health personnel including pharmacists to participate in the entire planning. Public health management during disasters requires modification and expansion of various health services and medical capabilities to counter a situation more effectively.

Role of Pharmacist In Disaster Management

Importance of pharmacists in disaster management: The importance of medication distribution and patient care during disasters is vital. Pharmacists offer accessibility that is unique among health care professionals as:

- Pharmacists work in a variety of public settings, including hospitals, drug, grocery, and retail stores, and nursing homes.

- The people in the community can reach pharmacists easily as compared to other health care professionals and they can provide public health services round the clock without appointments.

- Pharmacists often offer emergency care alternatives in case of staff shortage. Pharmacists have varying degrees of knowledge related to pathophysiological parameters, adverse drug reactions, drug interactions, drug administration, pharmacological concepts; etc makes them valuable for the affected patients in faraway places until any medical aid reaches them.

Activities of a pharmacist in PPRR cycle of disaster management

Disaster medicine is the study and collaborative application of various health disciplines to the **prevention, preparedness, response, and recovery**, arising from a disaster. This must be achieved in cooperation with all disciplines of health systems involved in disaster management.

Pharmacists are the most common health care professionals. The pharmacist's centralized position in the community makes them valuable **during disasters to provide healthcare continuity.** Apart from dispensing medicine, pharmacists have proven to be an accessible resource for health and medication information. There are many functions of public health that can benefit from pharmacists' unique expertise including pharmacotherapy, access to care, and prevention services.

Prevention: Preventing future threats of disaster and/or minimizing the damaging effects of unavoidable threats. For prevention pharmacists are involved in:

- Optimizing medication supplies for chronic disease management.

- Administer vaccinations.

- Educate the public on reducing the spread of communicable diseases/infections.

- Ensuring patients are aware of their increased risk of adverse health outcomes in a disaster.

- Tailored 'point of care' messaging to chronic disease patients.

Preparedness includes a group of activities designed to minimize the impact of disasters on people's life. The activities are identification, assessment, and planning management of disaster-related risks. The pharmacists need to be prepared for:

➢ Ensuring an uninterrupted supply of essential medications in a disaster.

➢ Establishing systems to maintain cold chain lines.

➢ Being a part of the local community disaster management teams to coordinate pharmaceutical response

➢ Knowing how to access pharmaceutical stockpiles if necessary.

➢ Being a part of local/state/national disaster preparedness health meetings for providing medication management advice.

Response: Response work includes any actions taken in the midst of or immediately following an emergency, including efforts to save lives and prevent further death and disability. The activities include:

➢ Dispense medications and other necessary medication-related items to affected members of the community (prescription, over-the-counter medications, inhalers).

➢ Counseling patients on how to use and take medications.

➢ Coordinating logistics of medications and medical supplies for patients with chronic diseases.

➢ Providing emergency medication supply refills for up to 30 days during the declared disaster.

➢ Assisting with the release and allocation of national stock piles if required in a pandemic or emergency.

➢ Rationing limited supplies of medications.

➢ Develop a list of at-risk patients in their community.

➢ Maintain systems and processes for the reconciliation and security of controlled drugs (e.g. morphine, codeine etc).

➢ Prescribing and administering vaccinations (e.g. tetanus, antidote/prophylaxis following state public health disaster protocols).

➢ Maintain media liaison on medication issues.

➢ Decide on the appropriateness of donated medications and other supplies.

➢ Institute cardiopulmonary resuscitation (CPR), providing wound care and first aid for minor ailments.

4. Recovery: This process pertains to the restoration of infrastructure and other facilities, and psychological support. It includes:

➢ Re-establish normal stock levels, and destroy contaminated stock appropriately.

➢ Restock emergency/disaster kits for the next disaster event.

➢ Check on the health needs of the local community.

➢ Identify and prioritize vulnerable patients in the local community.

➢ Restore order to patient records and drug records.

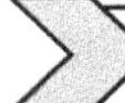

CHAPTER 7

Pharmacoeconomics

7.1 Pharmacoeconomics

Pharmacoeconomics is a branch of health economics that is related to patients, society, the economy and drug therapy. **'Pharmacoeconomics is defined as the science of measuring costs and outcomes associated with the use of pharmaceuticals in health care delivery.**

Its objective is to improve public health by making appropriate decisions when selecting alternative therapies and health care services. It focuses on the costs (inputs) and consequences (outcomes) of their use.

The goals of pharmacoeconomics are

1. To determine which healthcare alternative provides the best health care outcome in terms of money spent.

2. To improve the allocation of resources for pharmaceutical products and services.

Need for Pharmacoeconomics

1. **For Patients:** To find the optimal therapy at the lowest price

2. **For Industry:** To decide among specific research and development alternatives.

3. **For Government:** To determine program benefits and prices paid.

4. **In the Private sector:** To design insurance benefit coverage.

5. **For Pharmacists:** To make better and more informed decisions regarding products and services they provide.

Pharmacoeconomics Evaluation: Pharmacoeconomics research identifies measures and compares the costs (resources consumed) and consequences (clinical, economic, and, humanistic outcomes) of pharmaceutical products and services.

Economic efficiency is the ratio of costs divided by the outcomes. When comparing resources, the drug giving the most favorable outcomes at the lowest cost will be favored.

A. **Costs (Inputs):** The costs of medicines and health care services are rising day by day. In a country like India, a significant number of people live below the poverty line and have diverse health care needs. They cannot afford appropriate healthcare services as these resources are not easily accessible and affordable to many patients. Pharmacoeconomic evaluation plays an important role in finding the optimal therapy at the lowest price and determining the delivery of reasonable and cost-effective health services.

Costs are the resources consumed by the illness and by its treatment. Therefore, costs have to be measured under real-life conditions.

Table 7.1 Different types of costs

Direct Costs (Directly related to the treatment)	Indirect Costs (Related to loss of productivity due to illness)	Intangible Costs (Related to impairments of the quality of life)
➢ Prescription medications, self-medications ➢ Diagnosis and treatment of side effects and complications, ➢ Consultation of the doctor, ➢ Diagnostic investigations, ➢ Costs for hospital and nursing-home treatment. ➢ Transportation, ➢ Informal care by relatives.	➢ Absenteeism from job/work, ➢ Premature pensioning because of disability ➢ Premature death (e.g: by suicide) ➢ Concerning psychiatric disorders ➢ costs of violence and crime also have to be considered	➢ Impaired quality of life of the patients, their relatives, and friends involved in the care.

B. Outcomes (consequences): These are the possible end results of a particular treatment. Outcomes depend on the effectiveness of the treatment under the influence of all the variables in real life. Pharmacotherapy decisions traditionally depended solely on clinical outcomes like safety and efficacy, but pharmacoeconomics teaches us that there are three basic outcomes to be considered clinical, economic, and humanistic in drug therapy.

The **'ECHO'** model of pharmacoeconomics research evaluates **E**conomic (Cost efficiency), **C**linical (treatment effectiveness), and **H**umanistic (Impact on the healthcare system, individual, and society) outcomes.

Clinical outcomes are related to the overall well-being of the patient. Examples are:

➢ Positive outcomes: Drug efficacy measures, cure, comfort and survival

➢ Negative outcomes: Adverse drug reaction and treatment failure.

Economic outcomes are related to saving, cost avoidance, expense and best utilization of resources in terms of money.

Economic evaluations

➢ Partial economic evaluations

➢ Cost consequence analysis (CCA) or Cost outcome analysis (COA)

➢ Cost-of-illness (COI) evaluation

Full economic evaluations

➢ Cost Minimization Analysis (CMA)

➢ Cost Benefit Analysis (CBA)

➢ Cost Effectiveness Analysis (CEA)

➢ Cost-Utility analysis (CUA)

Humanistic outcomes are related to the physical, social, and emotional aspects of a patient's well-being.

Humanistic evaluation methods are:

➢ Health Regulated Quality of Life (HRQOL)

➢ Patient Preferences

➢ Patient Satisfaction

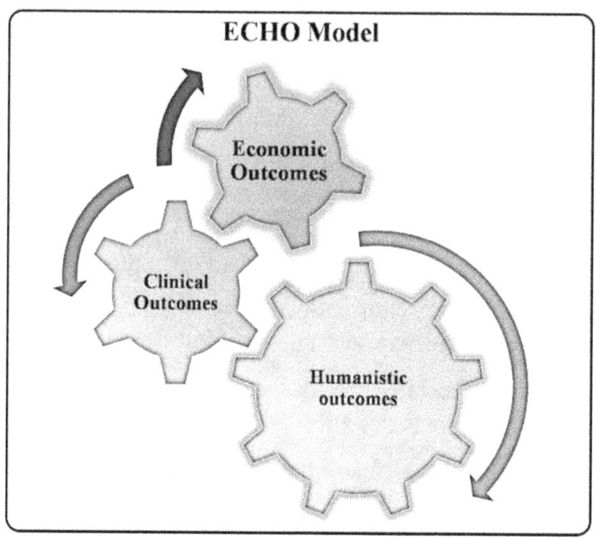

Figure 7.1 The ECHO model

Table 7.2 Description of important Pharmacoeconomic methodologies

S. No.	Method	Description	Application
1	**Cost-of-illness evaluation (COI)**	Estimates the cost of a disease on a defined population	Use to provide a baseline to compare prevention/treatment options a gainst a disease.
2	**Cost-minimization analy sis (CMA)**	Finds the least expensive cost alternative	Use when benefits are the same.
3	**Cost-benefit analysis (CBA)**	Measures benefit in monetary units and compute a net gain.	Can compare programs with different objectives.
4	**Cost-effectiveness analys is (CEA)**	Compares alternatives with therapeutic effects measured in physical units; computes a cost-effectiveness ratio	Can compare drugs/programs that differ in clinical outcomes and use the same unit of benefit
5	**Cost-utility analysis (CUA)**	Can compare drugs/programs that differ in clinical outcomes and use the same unit of benefit	Compare medications/programs with serious side effects or those producing reductions in morbidity
6	**Quality of life (QOL)**	Physical, social, and emotional aspects of the patient's well-being that are relevant and important to the patient	Examines drug effects in areas not covered by laboratory or physiologic measurements

Significance of Pharmacoeconomics

➢ Pharmacoeconomic methods are utilized to assist physicians, hospitals, insurance companies, patients, and healthcare professionals in making important decisions as to what drug therapies should be chosen.

➢ Used to determine which drug should be included in the formulary by choosing the most effective treatment at the lowest price.

➢ Can be utilized to create clinical guidelines for physicians that will assist them in prescribing the most efficient drug.

➢ In addition to drug versus drug decisions, pharmacoeconomics allows us to make decisions between drugs versus surgery and drugs versus watchful waiting based on the effectiveness of the treatment and the cost.

➢ An essential tool in therapeutic decision-making.

Applications of Pharmacoeconomics

➢ Allows the pharmacy practitioners and administrators to make better and more informed decisions regarding the products and services they provide.

➢ Makes the best use of limited resources.

➢ Improves the allocation of resources for pharmaceutical products and services.

➢ Determines which healthcare alternatives provide the best healthcare outcome in terms of money spent by comparing the costs and benefits of available therapeutic options, and treatment services and helps in making the best choice.

➢ Assesses the value of a new agent, helps to decide which drug to develop, and estimates and understands the full impact of a new therapy.

➢ Justifies drug policy decisions, treatment guidelines, and the addition of new clinical services.

➢ It also helps in establishing accountability that the claims by a manufacturer regarding a drug are justified.

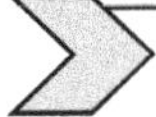

7.2   Health Insurance

Insurance is an arrangement by which a company or a state or government undertakes to provide a guarantee of compensation for the specified loss, damage, illness, or death in return for the payment of a specified insurance premium.

Health Insurance: It is a type of insurance that covers medical expenses that arise due to an illness. These expenses could be related to hospitalization costs, cost of medicines, or doctor consultation fees. The premium amount is calculated based on age, gender, health status, lifestyle, and other factors.

Terminology related to Health Insurance

Insurance premium: An amount of money paid periodically or as an installment to maintain the insurance coverage as specified by the company in an insurance policy. Failure to pay the premium may result in the cancellation of the policy and a loss of coverage. Insurance premiums are paid for the policy that covers health care, auto, home, and life.

Provider: any person (i.e., doctor, nurse, dentist) or institution (i.e., hospital or clinic) that provides medical care.

Rider: coverage options that enable you to expand your basic insurance plan for an additional premium. A common example is a maternity rider.

Claim: a request by a plan customer, or a plan customer's health care provider, for the insurance company to pay for medical services.

Importance of Health Insurance

➢ Health insurance coverage helps people get timely medical care and improves their lives and health outcomes.

➢ The insured person receives preventive and screening services on regular basis. For uninsured persons, diseases are more likely to be diagnosed at a later stage of illness, when treatment is less effective.

➢ Uninsured people and their families suffer financial burdens. They sometimes do not benefit from a private health plan or public program discounts.

➢ Having health coverage is associated with better health-related outcomes.

➢ An insured person can expand coverage at some additional costs for added services.

Services provided via Health Insurance Schemes: The health care providers keep on changing the facilities they provide from time to time. Some of these are:

Cashless facility

➢ For all kinds of **surgeries.**

➢ **Daycare procedures** like chemotherapy, cataract surgery dialysis.

➢ **In-patient department admissions:** 24 hr hospital admission for medical illness road traffic accidents, and trauma, it includes all expenses like IPD charges, pharmacy charges, and investigation charges. Under some of the schemes delivery and caesarian charges are also covered.

➢ **Other facilities:** Pre-hospitalization and post-hospitalization charges (medicines, physiotherapy etc.) are also covered in certain schemes.

Government Health Insurance Schemes in India

A Government health insurance scheme is a State or Central Government powered initiative for its citizens. Such insurance policies offer a sizeable sum of insurance at a very low-priced annual premium.

Benefits of Government Health Insurance Plans

1. Policies are offered at a low price.

2. Encourages people below the poverty line to avail insurance.

3. Ensures the poor people have some sort of insurance cover.

4. The government-initiated policies help policyholders to feel assured.

5. Inclusion of Government as well as Private hospitals for better healthcare.

Following are the Centre Government Health Insurance Schemes in India:

1. Ayushman Bharat Yojna:

➢ It was initiated on the recommendations of the National Health Policy with an aim to provide Universal Health Coverage for the people of India.

➢ The two components related to this scheme are Health and Wellness Centres (HWC) and Pradhan Mantri Jan Arogya Yojana (PM-JAY) for the poor.

➢ It offers a health cover of rupees 5 lakhs per family on an annual basis, and the payable premium is rupees 30.

➢ 150000 HWCs have been created in order to ensure better healthcare for the people.

2. Central Government Health Scheme (CGHS):

➢ The scheme was initiated six decades before by the Indian Government.

➢ It provides coverage to approximately 35 lakh employees and pensioners of the Central Government including Supreme Court judges and Certain Railway Board employees, etc.

➢ Hospitalization, as well as domiciliary care are covered.

3. Employees State Insurance Scheme (ESI):

➢ This provides financial cover to the employees in case of illness, disability, or death faced by insured workers/employees

➢ Injuries and deaths due to working conditions are covered under this scheme.

➢ More than 7 lakh factories are a part of this scheme.

4.   Pradhan Mantri Suraksha Bima Yojana:

➢ This scheme offers accident insurance to people (aged 18 to 70) in India having a bank account.

➢ The premium of Rs.12 gets debited automatically from the insured person's bank account.

➢ This policy provides an annual cover of 1 lakh for partial disability and 2 lakhs for total disability/death.

5. Rashtriya Swasthya Bima Yojana:

➢ This scheme is initiated by the Indian Government's Ministry of Labour and Employment.

➢ It provides coverage to workers in the unorganized sector and those below the poverty line.

➢ The cover also extends to their family (maximum of five members).

6.   Universal Health Insurance Scheme:

➢ In India, the benefits can be availed by the poorest of the poor in the age group of 5 to 70 years.

➢ It offers individual as well as covering hospitalization, accident, and disability.

➢ The premium depends on the size of the family. Those falling under the poverty line need to show proper documentation to avail the policy.

7. Aam Aadmi Bima Yojana:

➢ Aam Aadmi Bima Yojana is meant for a family head or an earning member of one's family involved in carpentry, fishing, handloom, weaving, etc.

➢ Before 2013, there were two policies of similar nature, AABY and Janashree Bima Yojana (JBY). After 2013, JBY was merged with AABY.

➢ The premium for 30000 rupees insurance policy is 200 rupees for a year.

8. Pradhan Mantri Garib Kalyan Package Insurance: Short-term plans proposed during health emergencies like COVID-19 pandemic for frontline warriors.

Table 7.3 Health Insurance Schemes in different States of India

S.No	State	Name of the scheme	Important features of the scheme
1	Kerala	Awaz Health Insurance Scheme:	➤ Provides coverage of Rs.2 lakh laborers (aged 18 to 60) in case of death by accident. ➤ Health Insurance cover is Rs.15000,
		Karunya Health Scheme (2012)	➤ It is a Critical Illness plan for the poor and covers major diseases such as cancer, kidney ailments, heart-related medical issues, etc. ➤ Aadhaar Card and appropriate income certificate are needed for this scheme.
2	Rajasthan	Rajasthan's Chiranjeevi Yojana	➤ Annual cashless health insurance cover of Rs 5 lakh to every family in the State. ➤ Covers1576 treatment packages for various diseases. ➤ Covers medical expenses for 5 days pre and 15 days post- hospitalization. ➤ Registration fee for this scheme is Rs 850 which is 50% of the annual premium. ➤ Free registration for people covered under the National Food Security Act, Socio-Economic Caste Census, small and marginal farmers, contractual workers.
3	Odisha	Odisha's Biju Swastya Kalyan Yojana	➤ Free health services for all irrespective of income, status or residence in all government hospitals. ➤ Annual Health coverage of Rs 5 lakh / family and Rs 7 lakh for the women members of the family covers 4036 treatment packages providing free of cost health services that include medicines, diagnostics, dialysis, free Cancer chemotherapy, free OT, free I.C.U, free in-patient admission.
4	West Bengal	West Bengal's Swasthya Sathi Yojana	➤ Provides Cashless, smart card based health cover of Rs. 5 lakh /year/ family for secondary and tertiary care. ➤ 2092 treatment packages are available in the scheme, no cap on the family size, also covers all pre-existing diseases,
		West Bengal Health Scheme	➤ Also called as Cashless Medical Treatment Scheme ➤ Provides health cover of Rs. 1 lakh. to an individual and his family members for OPD and all services except cosmetic surgeries and non-emergency procedures.

Table 7.3 *contd...*

S.No	State	Name of the scheme	Important features of the scheme
5	Tamilnadu	Chief Minister's Comprehensive Insurance Scheme	➢ This scheme promoted by Tamil Nadu Government in association with United India Insurance Company Ltd. is for the people of Tamil Nadu earning less than Rs. 75000/ year. ➢ It is a family floater plan designed for quality health care. ➢ Approximately 1027 procedures are covered under this insurance scheme. ➢ The hospitalization expenses up to Rs. 5 lakhs in selected government and private hospitals can be claimed in a single claim.
6	Punjab	Bhagat Puran Singh Sehat Bima Yojna	➢ Provides coverage to 37 lakh BPL families
7	Chhattisgarh	CM's SwasthyaBima Yojna	➢ Provides health coverage to each family of the state by issuing insurance of Rs 60 only. ➢ 60 lakh cards have been issued to date.
8	Maharashtra	Mahatma Jyotiba Phule Jan Arogya Yojana	➢ This policy is initiated by the Government of Maharashtra. ➢ Rajiv Gandhi Jeevandayee Arogya Yojana was renamed as in the year 2017. ➢ Farmers and people below and around the poverty line are eligible for this scheme. ➢ Provides health coverage of Rs. 150000 per family.
9	Gujrat	Mukhyamantri Amrutum Yojana:	➢ Lower middle-class families and those living below the poverty line are eligible for this cover. ➢ Provides cover of Rs. 3 lakhs/ year /family for various treatments in govt, private hospitals, trust-based and Grant-in-Aid hospitals.
10	Telangana	Telangana State Government – Employees and Journalists Health Scheme	➢ The scheme provides cashless treatment to its existing and retired employees and journalists ➢ Beneficiaries can avail of cashless treatment in hospitals listed under the scheme even in an emergency.
		Telangana's Aarogyasri Yojana	➢ Scheme covers BPL families with a coverage of 2.5 lakhs/ family free of cost. ➢ The entire premium is paid by the Government. ➢ All pre-existing diseases covered ➢ Coverage of 949 different treatment package for patients along with free food and transportation.

Table 7.3 *contd…*

S.No	State	Name of the scheme	Important features of the scheme
11	Andhra Pradesh	Dr YSR Aarogyasri Health Care Trust Andhra Pradesh State Government	The Andhra Pradesh Government along with the Dr. YSR Aarogyasri Trust, which works for health care, runs four health welfare schemes for its people. The schemes are: ➢ This scheme is dedicated to the welfare of the poor. ➢ This scheme is for journalists and it offers cashless treatment in case of listed procedures. ➢ This scheme is for the benefit of state government employees.
12	Karnataka	Yeshasvini Health Insurance Scheme:	➢ It is for farmers and peasants associated with a cooperative society. Enrollment is done with the help of Cooperative societies. ➢ The scheme extends its benefits to the family members of the main beneficiary as well. ➢ Covers 800 procedures (Orthopaedic, Neurology, Angioplasty, etc.) as per this insurance policy through network hospitals.

Health Spendings

Individual health insurance: Health insurance plans are purchased by individuals to cover themselves and their families against illnesses and diseases. These plans are different from group plans, which are offered by employers to cover all of their employees.

With an increase in age, healthcare needs also change. So while buying a healthcare plan it is advisable to anticipate annual healthcare costs and then decide on the coverage and annual premium. The premium payment for the healthcare plan is not an out-of-pocket expense.

Out-of-Pocket expenses: Out-of-pocket expenses refer to the portion of the bill that the insurance company doesn't cover and that the individual must pay on their own. Sometimes these expenses exceed anticipated amounts.

Out-of-pocket healthcare expenses include **deductibles, copays, and coinsurance.**

Deductible: The amount of money you must pay each year to cover eligible medical expenses before your insurance policy starts paying.

Copayment: One of the ways you share in your medical costs. You pay a flat fee for certain medical expenses while the rest is paid by the insurance company.

Coinsurance: The amount you pay to share the cost of covered services after your deductible has been paid. The coinsurance rate is usually a percentage. For example, if the insurance company pays 80% of the claim, you pay 20%.

Out-of-pocket maximum: An annual out-of-pocket maximum is the amount a policyholder must pay for healthcare, excluding the premium. After the policyholder reaches that amount, the insurance plan covers all eligible healthcare expenses for the year.

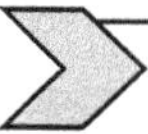 ## 7.3   Health Maintenance Organizations (HMO)

In countries, where medical expenses are high, medical insurance is a must. Medical insurance allows patients to see doctors when sick without paying the full cost. Managed care organizations (MCO) coordinate the finance and delivery of healthcare to insured individuals. These organizations have a network of doctors and healthcare professionals that provide care with an aim to control costs without compromising quality

The most important medical managed care organization is Health Maintenance Organisation (**HMO**). It is a health insurance plan that is offered by insurance companies in the United States.

HMO is an organization of physicians or other healthcare professionals that provides a broad and nearly complete range of healthcare services on a prepaid basis.

Health Maintenance Organization (HMO)

➢ HMO is a type of managed care organization that creates and maintains a network of patients and doctors and arranges managed care on a prepaid basis.

➢ HMO provides comprehensive health care (coverage) to a voluntarily enrolled person on payment of a fixed price. Members pay fixed, periodic (usually monthly/ annually) fees directly to the HMO and in return receive healthcare services from the HMO's network of providers (physicians, hospitals, and other healthcare providers).

➢ The doctors and practitioners are paid on annual basis, whether the patients avail the services or not.

Working of HMO

HMOs contract directly with physicians, hospitals, and other healthcare providers. Most HMOs cover basic health services such as physician services, inpatient/outpatient hospital services, emergency visits, referral services, laboratory services, and more.

➢ HMO plan provides health coverage for enrolling for a prepaid fixed premium that is called capitation. Network provider offers their services at discounted rates.

➢ These plans provide a larger menu of services than those provided in the traditional fee-for-service plans.

➢ In this, a network of doctors, patients, specialists, hospitals, and test centers is maintained. The doctors-medical practitioners under contract are paid on an annual basis whether the patients avail the services or not.

➢ HMO is considered to be more restrictive when it comes to medical care as the patient can only pick from a selected list of medical providers that are part of the organization's network and are contracted with them.

➢ The enrolled patient has to select a primary care physician (PCP) from the network. The patients are supposed to see PCP first.

➢ In case the patient wishes to see a specialist they would require a referral from their PCP.

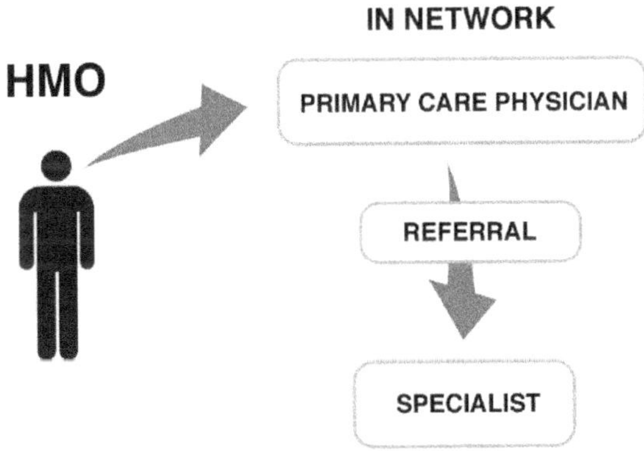

Figure 7.2 Working of HMO

Primary Care Physician (PCP)

➢ PCPs are generally **family doctors**, internal medicine doctors, pediatricians, general practitioners, and the **patient's case managers.**

➢ The PCPs are **the gatekeepers** that provide, coordinate and manage all health care needs of members.

➢ PCP will be responsible for mapping and charting the patient's **whole medical care.**

➢ PCPs **provide and revise prescriptions.**

➢ If the patient needs to see a specialist he would require a **referral /approval of referral** from his PCP to visit a specialist that is on the network

➢ If a primary care physician leaves the network patient will need to change doctor.

Advantages of HMOs:

1. Cost (Premium) is comparatively cheaper and affordable than other network providers.

2. Cover more healthcare services than those available through other traditional healthcare plans.

3. Provides ready access to healthcare, early detection, and treatment of disease and helps maintain better health.

4. Beneficial for people who only need basic medical care such as essential checkups and immunization.

5. Usually, one doctor for most of the services is there. The PCP is more like a personal doctor and there are no restrictions on the number of primary care visits.

6. Drug costs are kept low generally requiring only a small copayment and both generic and brand name drugs are available.

7. Usually, patients will not be required to submit claims to the insurance company; it is done by the providers

Disadvantages of HMOs:

1. It provides major medical treatment of illness including pharmacy coverage only when using in-network providers. Patients would be fully responsible for paying doctors that are not under the network.

2. Need a referral from primary care physician to consult a specialist for obtaining certain services.

3. In certain cases, prescription drugs are not covered.

4. Emergency treatments are not covered.

5. Doctors under this plan may become careless with their patients as they get paid either way.

Appendix

Logos of Important National Health Programs of India

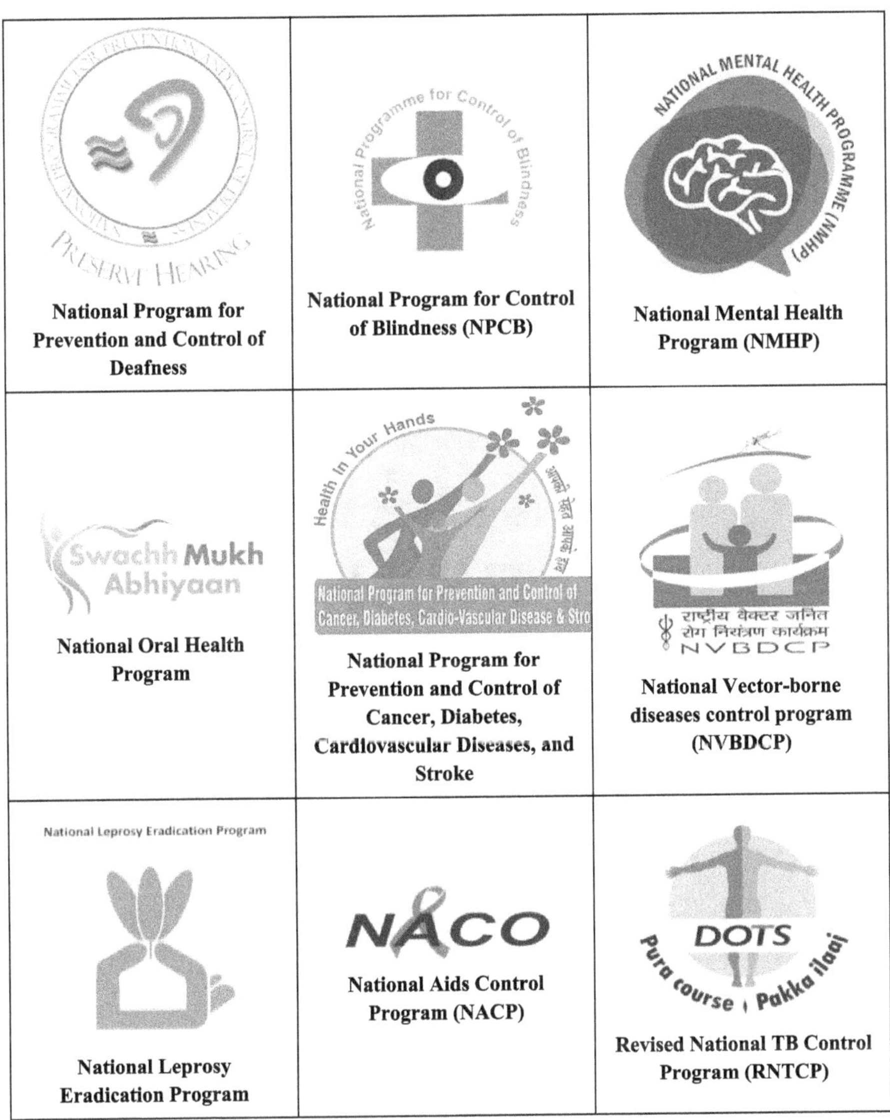

National Program for Prevention and Control of Deafness	National Program for Control of Blindness (NPCB)	National Mental Health Program (NMHP)
National Oral Health Program	National Program for Prevention and Control of Cancer, Diabetes, Cardiovascular Diseases, and Stroke	National Vector-borne diseases control program (NVBDCP)
National Leprosy Eradication Program	National Aids Control Program (NACP)	Revised National TB Control Program (RNTCP)

Table *contd....*

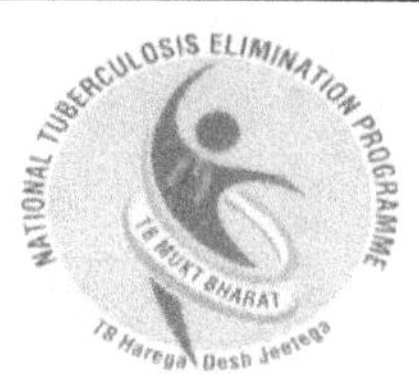

National Tuberculosis Elimination Program

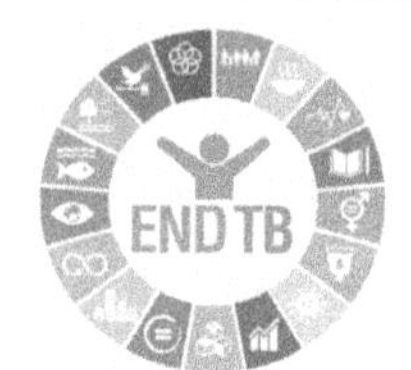

National Strategic Plan for TB elimination

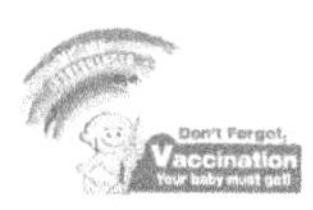

Intensified Mission Indra dhanush

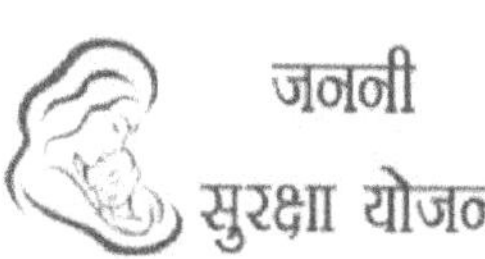

Janani Suraksha Yojana (JSY)

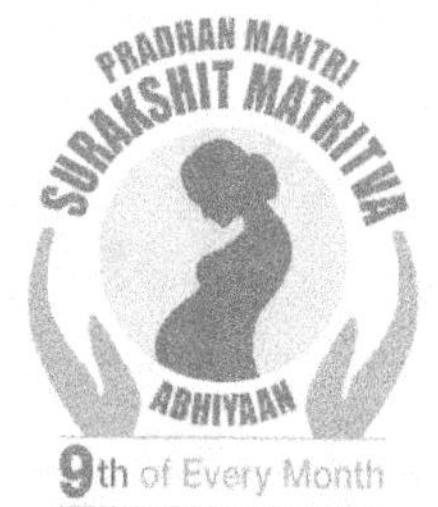

Pradhan Mantri Surakshit Matritva Abhiyan (PMSMA)

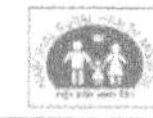

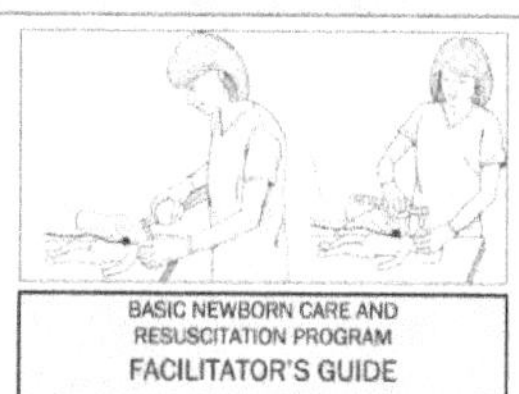

Navjaat Shishu Suraksha Karyakram (NSSK)

Family Planning Program

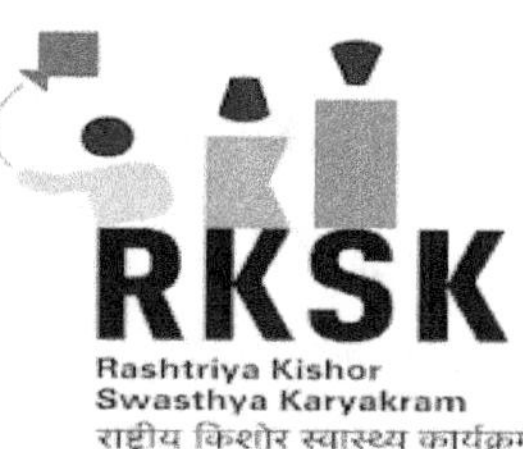

Rashtriya Kishor Swasthya Karyakram (RKSK)

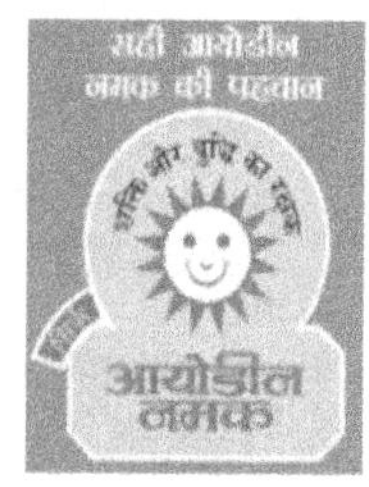

National Iodine Deficiency Disorders Control Program

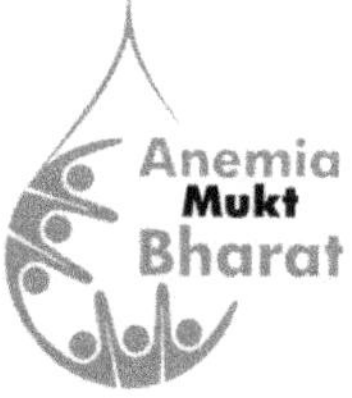

Intensified National iron plus initiative (I-NIPI) for Anaemia Control

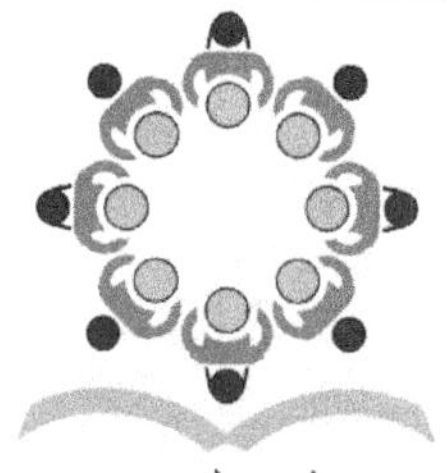

Mid-day Meal Scheme

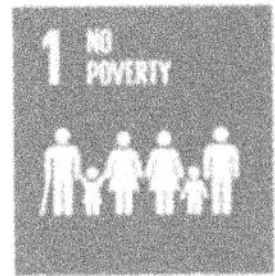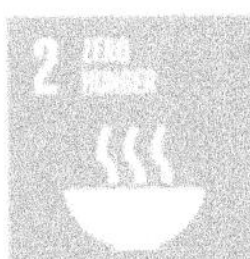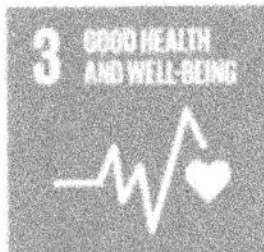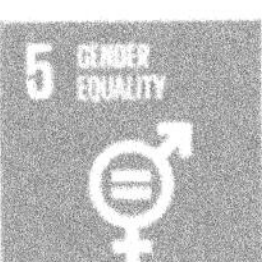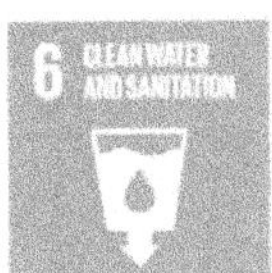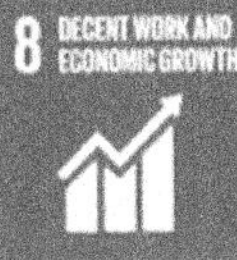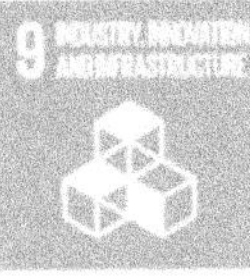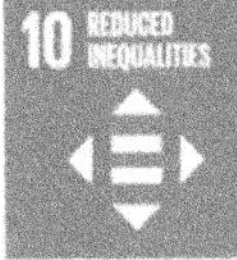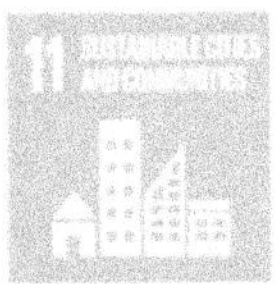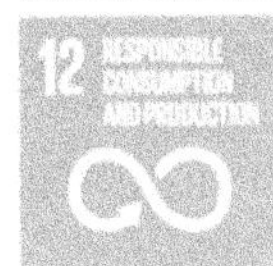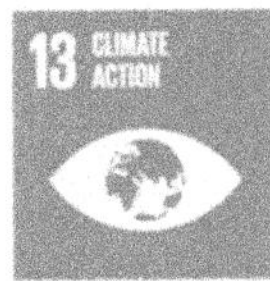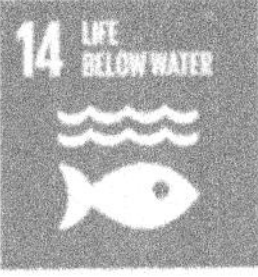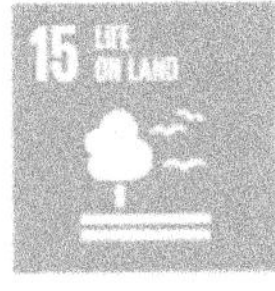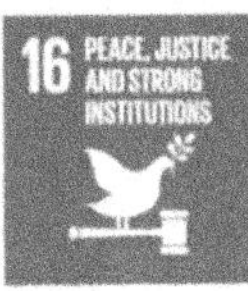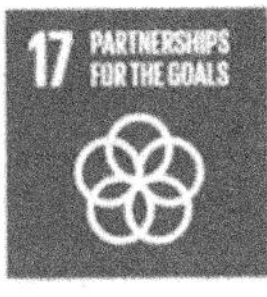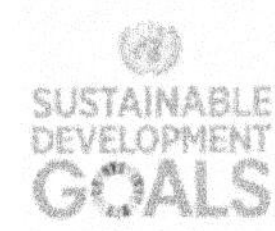

SUSTAINABLE DEVELOPMENT GOALS
1 NO POVERTY
2 ZERO HUNGER
3 GOOD HEALTH AND WELL-BEING
4 QUALITY EDUCATION
5 GENDER EQUALITY
6 CLEAN WATER AND SANITATION
7 AFFORDABLE AND CLEAN ENERGY
8 DECENT WORK AND ECONOMIC GROWTH
9 INDUSTRY, INNOVATION AND INFRASTRUCTURE
10 REDUCED INEQUALITIES
11 SUSTAINABLE CITIES AND COMMUNITIES
12 RESPONSIBLE CONSUMPTION AND PRODUCTION
13 CLIMATE ACTION
14 LIFE BELOW WATER
15 LIFE ON LAND
16 PEACE, JUSTICE AND STRONG INSTITUTIONS
17 PARTNERSHIPS FOR THE GOALS
SUSTAINABLE DEVELOPMENT GOALS

www.ingramcontent.com/pod-product-compliance
Lightning Source LLC
Chambersburg PA
CBHW050744150726
48196CB00003B/356